The Complete Guide

Providing Telephone Triage and Advice in a Family Practice

During Office Hours and/or After Hours

Steven R. Poole, MD

Clinical Professor of Family Medicine

Professor and Vice Chair, Department of Pediatrics

University of Colorado School of Medicine

Medical Director, The Children's Hospital Regional Health Care Network, Denver, CO

Cofounder and Administrative Director, Children's Hospital After-Hours Telephone Care Program

Founding Chairperson, American Academy of Pediatrics Section on Telephone Care

AAP Department of Marketing and Publications Staff

Maureen DeRosa, Director, Department of Marketing and Publications

Mark Grimes, Director, Division of Product Development
Diane Beausoleil, Senior Product Development Editor
Kate Simone, Electronic Publishing Manager

Sandi King, Director, Division of Publishing and Production Services
Kate Larson, Manager, Editorial Services
Jason Crase, Editorial Specialist
Leesa Levin-Doroba, Manager, Print Production Services
Linda Diamond, Manager, Graphic Design
Peg Mulcahy, Graphic Designer

Jill Ferguson, Director, Division of Marketing and Sales
Linda Smessaert, Manager, Publication and Program Marketing

Natalie Arndt, Department Coordinator

Library of Congress Control Number: 2003101674

ISBN: 1-58110-116-3

MA0243

Contributors

Barton D. Schmitt, MD, FAAP
Professor of Pediatrics, University of Colorado School of Medicine
Medical Director, The Children's Hospital After-Hours Telephone Care Program, Denver, CO

Sanford M. Melzer, MD, FAAP
Associate Professor of Pediatrics, University of Washington School of Medicine
Vice President, Regional and Ambulatory Care
Children's Hospital & Regional Medical Center, Seattle, WA

Andrew R. Hertz, MD, FAAP
Medical Director, Rainbow Advice Center
Rainbow Babies and Children's Hospital
Assistant Clinical Professor of Pediatrics
Case Western Reserve University, Cleveland, OH

Elaine Donoghue, MD, FAAP
Clinical Associate Professor
Department of Pediatrics, UMDNJ-Robert Wood Johnson Medical School
Saint Peter's University Hospital, New Brunswick, NJ

Dipti Amin, MD, FAAP
Clinical Associate Professor of Pediatrics at University of South Florida, School of Medicine
Medical Director of the On-Call Program at All Children's Hospital
Director of Medical Informatics
All Children's Hospital, St Petersburg, FL

Hanna B. Sherman, MD, FAAP
Former Medical Director
Night Train Pediatrics (Call Center)
Children's Hospital, Boston, MA

Cecelia (Sissy) Tubb, RN, CPN, CACN
Manager, OU Medical Center Call Center
Oklahoma University Medical Center, Tulsa, OK

Reviewers

Steven Thorson, MD, FAAFP
Family Physician in Private Practice
Ft Collins, CO

Jeffrey J. Cain, MD, FAAFP
Assistant Professor, Department of Family Medicine
University of Colorado School of Medicine
Chief of Family Medicine, The Children's Hospital, Denver, CO

Barton D. Schmitt, MD, FAAP
Professor of Pediatrics, University of Colorado School of Medicine
Medical Director, The Children's Hospital After-Hours Telephone Care Program, Denver, CO

Hanna B. Sherman, MD, FAAP
Former Medical Director
Night Train Pediatrics (Call Center)
Children's Hospital, Boston, MA

A. D. Jacobson, MD, FAAP
Chair, Section on Ambulatory and Practice Management
American Academy of Pediatrics
Private Practice Pediatrician, Phoenix, AZ

Alane Hall, RN, BSN
Triage Manager
Aurora Pediatric Associates, Aurora, CO

Andrew R. Hertz, MD, FAAP
Medical Director, Rainbow Advice Center
Rainbow Babies and Children's Hospital
Assistant Clinical Professor of Pediatrics
Case Western Reserve University, Cleveland, OH

Teresa Hegarty, RN, BSN
System Coordinator
The Children's Hospital After-Hours Telephone Care Program, Denver, CO

Table of Contents

Introduction

A recent study conducted on telephone care in selected Colorado family practices during 2002 compared call volume with studies from earlier decades and showed that calls to family practices seeking clinical care by telephone (non-visit care) are increasing. Practices in the study handled from 15,000 to 17,000 telephone calls per year (on average 275-325 calls per week) per each family physician in the practice. Between 2,500 and 3,000 of those telephone calls (per family physician in the practice) involved clinical care. More than 2,000 clinical calls per year (8-10 per day) per family physician were handled during office hours and another 500 to 750 clinical calls per family physician per year occurred after office hours. During office hours these calls for non-visit care represented approximately 25% of all clinical patient contacts; after hours, they represented approximately 80% of all clinical contacts.

Telephone care involves at least 4 types of clinical care.
- *Telephone triage and advice,* in which telephone care providers determine the degree of urgency of the patient's problem, select the most appropriate disposition (time, location, and provider to handle the problem), and provide advice on what steps the caller should take to care for the patient.
- *Telephone health information and education,* in which telephone care providers answer health or illness questions and provide information and teaching.
- *Follow-up of an office visit by telephone* to reassess the condition or progress after the patient has been assessed at a visit.
- *Case management by telephone* to provide ongoing information and advice in the management of a chronic problem.

Providing care over the telephone is quite difficult because there is less information on which to make clinical decisions than with face-to-face office visits. As a result, telephone care involves a high degree of medicolegal risk. Even though it involves a high degree of clinical decision making and increased medicolegal risk, it is usually not reimbursed. Therefore, it is very challenging for family practices to provide cost-effective, quality telephone care. By developing a highly organized system of telephone care provided by well-trained staff, a family practice can improve cost-efficiency; quality of care; caller, office staff, and physician satisfaction; and reduce medicolegal risk.

This manual describes the methods and steps involved in developing and maintaining an effective telephone care system in a family practice during and after office hours. Recommended methods have been developed and tested over the past 15 years in telephone triage and advice call centers nationwide and, in recent years, by many primary care practices in Colorado. Samples of documentation forms, job descriptions, policies and procedures, telephone care standards, performance evaluation forms, and quality improvement (QI) materials are provided in this manual. Readers are encouraged to adapt the sample forms for use in their own practices.

This manual outlines a comprehensive, ideal system for providing telephone care. The system works easiest and is most affordable in a practice of at least 8 physicians. A large proportion of family physicians practice in smaller groups; all physicians can take elements of this system, adapt them to their practices, and create a model that works for them.

Getting Started

We recommend developing a small team to plan and begin to implement the telephone care system (or change the existing system). This team should include a nurse to serve as telephone care manager, a physician (or mid-level practitioner) to serve as telephone care medical director, and an office or practice manager to oversee the business aspects of telephone care. In small practices there may not be an office manager, but the business perspective will be important in planning. The team should meet initially to determine the scope and objectives for telephone care in the practice. There are several tasks for each person to accomplish at the beginning, after which, the telephone care manager can oversee the day-to-day telephone activities with periodic consultation from the medical director and practice manager.

In our study of family practice telephone care in Colorado, we realized that in some busy family practices almost anyone might be in the position of providing telephone care at some point, including registered nurses, licensed practical nurses, medical assistants, health assistants (people who have not received formal nursing training), reception/scheduling staff, and even the staff in the business office. Although we suggest that only people with health care training provide telephone triage and advice, we realize that may not always be practical. With that in mind, everyone who provides any type of clinical care or information in the practice should read chapters 2 through 4, 6, 11, and 14; complete the entire training process; understand telephone care standards, policies, and procedures; be evaluated; and participate in the QI process and ongoing telephone care education. The recommended chapters have been developed with particular emphasis on often-neglected key elements of telephone care and are well suited for reading by a trainee.

Chapter 6 is the heart of this manual and deserves special mention. First, it offers an efficient, effective method for providing training in telephone care. Second, Chapter 6 guides you in defining the model call for telephone care in your practice, which is one of the most important steps in developing a quality, cost-effective telephone care system. The model call defines the content and organization of a telephone care call that best reflects your practice style and values. Also, by carefully defining the model call, you will improve the cost-effectiveness of telephone care. The model call, then, becomes the basis for training, job descriptions, performance evaluation, policies, education of callers, staffing, ongoing staff education, and QI processes. Planning the model call should be done early in the process by at least the 3-person leadership team and ideally should include several of the telephone care providers.

This manual was written as a means of sharing what has been learned in telephone triage and advice call centers that can be applied to telephone care in private family practices. This manual is not intended to present standards for telephone care in family practice. Resources for providing telephone care are limited and highly variable in practice. Each practice must decide which of the suggestions made in this manual are appropriate for the practice. We hope you will find this manual useful.

Acknowledgments

I am grateful to the many people who have contributed to my understanding of telephone care and to the preparation of this manual.

Neil Chisolm, MD, who was chair of family medicine during my 6 years as a faculty member in the Department of Family Medicine at the University of Colorado School of Medicine. He taught me what it means to be a family physician.

Barton Schmitt, MD, medical director of The Children's Hospital After-Hours Telephone Care Program, Denver, CO, has spent more time than anyone else in the world working to improve the state of telephone care guidelines, and he has contributed a great deal to my understanding of the processes of telephone triage and advice.

The nurses in The Children's Hospital After-Hours Telephone Care Program, as we have learned together how to provide quality telephone care over the past 15 years. I particularly appreciate what they have taught me about performance evaluation, policies, and training.

Alane Hall, RN, the nurse manager of telephone care for Aurora Pediatric Associates, CO. Alane provided invaluable advice and reality testing for the approaches recommended in this manual.

Teresa Hegarty, RN, a very experienced pediatric telephone care nurse who provided advice and editorial assistance.

The members of the Executive Committee and chairs of Standing Committees of the American Academy of Pediatrics Section on Telephone Care, as we worked together to address the needs of pediatric professionals who provide telephone care for children: *Hanna Sherman, MD; Sandy Melzer, MD; Drew Hertz, MD; Allison Kempe, MD; Tony Luberti, MD; Ben Gitterman, MD; Elaine Donoghue, MD; Dipti Amin, MD;* and *Larry Simmons, MD.*

Jeff Cain, MD, assistant professor of family medicine at the University of Colorado School of Medicine, and *Steven Thorson, MD,* family physician in Fort Collins, CO, for their review of and important contributions to the manual.

The contributors and reviewers, who brought a wealth of knowledge and expertise from a wide variety of settings to this endeavor.

The family physicians in Colorado, who have consistently advised me and helped me to conduct a variety of telephone care studies. A special thanks to the physicians and staff of the Aurora Family Medicine Center, CO.

Jeff Poole, for conducting the research on telephone care in family practice.

Diane Beausoleil, for editorial review of the manual.

Chapter 1

Planning the Telephone Care System and Assigning Responsibilities

Providing high-quality, cost-effective telephone care requires planning, organization, monitoring, and continuous improvement. The first step in developing a telephone care system is to assign 3 important roles for overseeing the planning and initial implementation of the system (or changing the existing system). The 3 roles include a nurse to serve as telephone care manager, a physician (or mid-level practitioner) to serve as telephone care medical director, and an office or practice manager to oversee the business aspects of telephone care. In small practices, there may not be an office manager, but the business perspective will be important in planning. These 3 people will meet in the beginning to determine the scope and objectives for telephone care in the practice. This planning team will define the preferred format for clinical calls (the model call), select and adapt telephone care guidelines, design or select documentation forms, create policies and procedures, determine performance standards, agree on a process for complaint resolution, develop a plan for quality assurance, and make decisions about charging for telephone care. The telephone care manager can then develop and organize forms and materials and oversee training, evaluation, and the day-to-day telephone activities with periodic consultation with the medical director and practice manager. Appendix A provides a list of each of the steps for developing a complete telephone care system.

Physicians' Role in Telephone Care

In the 1950s, physicians handled all clinical calls themselves. Today, physicians delegate telephone care to office staff. As a result, physicians need to develop new knowledge and skills to be able to effectively advise those who train and supervise the telephone care staff and assume specific tasks associated with telephone care oversight. (See Table 1-1.) Medical direction for the office telephone care system should be provided by the physician or mid-level practitioner with the greatest interest in telephone care. The initial time commitment during planning and start-up will range from 6 to 8 hours, and the ongoing involvement for a 5-person practice averages from 1 to 2 hours per month.

Role of the Telephone Care Manager

The telephone care manager will be involved in planning and responsible for overseeing day-to-day telephone care activities. Duties include selecting, training, and evaluating telephone care providers, developing telephone care policies and procedures, managing the quality improvement (QI) activities, overseeing ongoing telephone care education, and handling most of the complaint resolution activities. The telephone care manager should have the following credentials:

- Experience and skill in providing telephone triage and advice
- Previous ambulatory care experience
- Good communication and interpersonal skills

- An aptitude for teaching
- Supervisory experience or good potential
- Good customer relations skills

The 2 most important skills for telephone care providers are the ability to quickly and empathetically guide the caller through the appropriate questions and the ability to come to closure on the call (wrap up) in a timely fashion. It is helpful for the telephone care manager to have these skills well developed. These skills often are innate, but can be most easily developed in a primary care office, emergency department, or urgent care setting.

The telephone care manager should plan to read this entire manual to understand all of the potential components of a telephone care system. The telephone care manager also organizes, supervises, and coordinates all facets of the office telephone care program. The time required for these duties depends on the size of the practice. It can fit in with the other supervisory responsibilities of the practice head nurse or a mid-level practitioner. Some of these duties require consultation with the medical director, such as planning the model call, developing standards, selecting telephone care guidelines, developing documentation forms, evaluating performance, and coordinating QI activities. The duties are described in Table 1-2.

Duties of the Office (Business) Manager

The person who is responsible for fiscal planning, budgeting, and paying the bills for the practice will be most interested in chapters 16 through 19, which describe reimbursement, staffing, telephone care expenses, and cost reduction methods. Other chapters will be of interest to the office manager if that person participates in hiring and staff evaluation (chapters 7, 8, and 17). It also will be helpful for the office manager to participate in defining the model call (Chapter 6) and caller satisfaction standards (Chapter 11). The chapters on after-hours telephone care also may be of interest (chapters 20-23).

The office manager should participate in the planning process, periodically meet with the telephone care manager, and participate in the QI process (because the practice will need to balance quality of care with cost).

Table 1-1
Responsibilities of the Telephone Care Medical Director

Task	Frequency/Phase
Become knowledgeable about ways to reduce medicolegal risk.	Initially
Help design telephone care documentation forms.	Initially
Select and review telephone care guidelines and modify them to be compatible with office and community practice style.	Initially
Reassess and modify telephone care guidelines.	Annually
Participate in developing telephone care policies and procedures.	Initially
Participate in creating performance standards and training objectives.	Initially
Participate in evaluating telephone care staff.	Periodically
Respond to some of the caller complaints about telephone care.	As needed, ongoing
Participate in the telephone care quality improvement meetings, and provide regular outcomes feedback to the telephone care providers.	Monthly or quarterly
Provide feedback to telephone care providers about outcomes of providers' triage and advice.	Ongoing
Decide what to charge for telephone care, and negotiate with payers for reimbursement.	Initially and annually
Serve as a backup for telephone care providers.	Ongoing

Table 1-2
Responsibilities of the Telephone Care Manager

Task	Frequency/Phase
Develop performance standards and job descriptions.	Initially, as needed
Select telephone care providers.	Initially, as needed
Train telephone care providers.	Initially, as needed
Supervise continuing education of telephone care providers.	Regular meetings
Evaluate telephone care providers.	Regularly scheduled
Develop policies and procedures.	Initially, as needed
Coordinate staffing of telephone care providers.	Ongoing
Coordinate telephone care quality improvement activities.	Ongoing
Maintain supplies, materials, and telephone care work space.	Ongoing
Manage complaints about telephone care.	As needed
Oversee the collection of data on telephone care outcomes and caller satisfaction and implement changes as needed.	Ongoing
Serve as a knowledgeable resource for telephone care providers.	Ongoing
Communicate program changes.	As needed
Involve the telephone care medical director in decision making.	As needed
Review all documentation of after-hours calls that are handled by a call center or other call providers outside the practice.	Ongoing

Chapter 2

Medicolegal Risk Reduction

Why devote one of the first chapters of this book to the topic of medicolegal risk? Telephone care is one of the highest-risk activities for a family practice. The primary objective in telephone care must be to provide quality care in a cost-efficient manner without placing patients at risk. There are no published standards for telephone care in family practice, but many important lessons about quality of care can be learned from case law that has developed around telephone care in office practice.

It is essential for risk management that physicians understand that any medical advice provided by a practice employee over the telephone on which the caller may reasonably rely establishes a provider-patient relationship, is considered medical practice, and the physicians are legally responsible for that advice. Medicolegal risk for telephone care is high in family practice for several reasons, including incomplete history; inability to examine the patient; inability to appreciate nuances of communication, such as facial expressions; lack (or paucity) of documentation; increasing volume, acuity, and complexity of telephone care; and pressure from managed care and patients to reduce the number of office and emergency department visits.

Regardless of who in the office provides the telephone advice, and no matter what training they have received, the owner of the practice and the physician who is present or supervising are liable. When care is provided by a medical call center, the telephone care provider and supervising physician of the medical call center are liable, and the primary care physician has little or no liability, as long as the medical call center is reputable and was selected carefully. Case law in several states has indicated that when a nurse (eg, in a medical call center) who is providing telephone advice in turn receives even the slightest advice from a physician, the physician is liable. Therefore, the physician in this situation should be absolutely certain that the information received from the nurse is sufficient to render a decision; otherwise the physician should speak with the caller directly.

Principles of Medical Malpractice Case Law and Telephone Care

Because there are very few federal or state statutes addressing telephone care, current recommendations for reducing medicolegal risk are based on applying traditional principles of medical malpractice case law to telephone care. In a malpractice action, the plaintiff must prove (1) a duty to treat was established, (2) harm was done to the patient, (3) the provider's care did not meet community standards, and (4) the harm was the direct result of substandard or negligent treatment.

Duty to Treat

A duty to treat is assumed when a patient calls a physician or the physician's delegate (1) if an emergency exists (in which case the provider must assess and advise) or (2) when the provider begins to give advice (at that point the provider becomes responsible to provide a "complete response," and to do otherwise constitutes abandonment). If the caller perceives that an emergency exists, then it is an emergency (especially if there is a bad outcome). If a patient makes telephone contact with someone in his or her primary care practice about a problem that the patient feels is an emergency, there is a duty to handle that problem until the problem is resolved or another health care source accepts the duty to treat. Therefore, if a patient describes symptoms that require an urgent response, but the office receptionist fails to recognize the urgency of the problem and schedules an appointment for the next day, the practice is liable. If a patient attempts to reach the person on-call about an urgent problem, but the on-call person fails to call back, the determination of liability depends on (1) whether the practice made an explicit or implied commitment to be available by telephone at that time and (2) whether the on-call person made a reasonable, good-faith effort to provide the availability the practice said it would provide.

If a provider begins to advise and then becomes unsure, he or she cannot back out of his or her duty to treat. When a nurse consults a physician and the physician provides any advice, it becomes the physician's case. The duty to treat persists until the problem is resolved or another provider accepts that duty. Therefore, good follow-up is an important element of medicolegal risk reduction.

Harm to the Patient and Substandard or Negligent Care Delivered
The most common lawsuit relating to telephone care involves a serious medical condition for which the seriousness was not recognized at the time of the call and, therefore, medical care was delayed and serious injury occurred. Once the duty to treat is accepted, the 2 most important errors made in telephone care that lead to malpractice judgments are (1) not obtaining enough information to recognize the seriousness of the problem that subsequently results in harm to the patient or (2) not sufficiently documenting the telephone encounter to show that standard, quality care was delivered. Therefore, the 2 most important elements of risk reduction in telephone care are (1) a systematic, thorough assessment of the problem(s), in a manner that is consistent with community standard of care (ideally accomplished using well-accepted telephone triage and advice guidelines), and (2) complete documentation of the care provided. It is our understanding that some malpractice insurance carriers have recently begun to expect practices to document all calls and use telephone care guidelines.

All members of a practice should participate in a planning session in which they assess their telephone care system and adapt it to ensure it can appropriately respond to potential emergency situations. A practice should be able to meet the challenge of appropriately handling a case such as in the following example:

> A mother whose 18-month-old child has a low-grade fever and a
> rash calls at 8:30 am, but there are no appointments until 4:30 pm.
> The mother is unaware that her child's rash is petechial and has no
> idea of its importance. This particular child has meningococcemia
> and is destined to become hypotensive and unresponsive by 4:00 pm.

This is an example of a patient with a very serious illness that is not readily apparent unless the call is subjected to carefully organized clinical questions and an appointment system that can accommodate patients who need to be urgently worked into the office schedule. How will your office be sure that this patient is not missed? This manual offers methods to protect against this situation.

Specific Recommendations for Reducing Medicolegal Risk

Require All Telephone Care Providers to Use Guidelines

The most effective means to ensure that each telephone care call receives standard of care is to use standardized telephone care guidelines (Chapter 3). These are now readily available and when they are used appropriately, they are considered to represent standard of care.

Document All Calls to Some Extent, and Selected Calls Thoroughly

The extent to which one documents any medical encounter is always a balance between patient care and safety, efficiency, and liability. The telephone encounter is no different and all calls in which triage or advice occurs should be documented, no matter who handles the call. Minimum recommended documentation for telephone encounters is covered in Chapter 4. More detailed documentation may be necessary for telephone calls involving greater risk (eg, calls about complex problems, repeat calls, medication changes or prescriptions, angry callers or callers who do not agree with recommendations, any call in which patients are instructed to seek immediate medical care).

All telephone care documentation should be archived, preferably in the patient's chart. Using documentation forms with carbon copies or removable stickers are acceptable alternatives to written or dictated telephone care notes. It is acceptable, but least desirable, to keep documentation of phone calls in a call log and transfer calls related to changes in medical management or high legal risk issues into the patient chart.

Exclude Nonclinical Staff From Providing Telephone Triage and Advice

Interviews with jurors from malpractice cases involving telephone care have indicated that nurses are considered appropriate providers of telephone triage and advice. They are somewhat less supportive of medical assistants (MAs) and even less supportive of health assistants who have no formal clinical training. The most common telephone care lawsuit involves reception/scheduling staff not recognizing the urgency of the underlying problem when a caller requests an appointment. To reduce this medicolegal risk, reception/scheduling staff (who do not have clinical training) should be encouraged to use the following approach. They may ask if the caller wants an appointment. If the caller does, the reception/scheduling staff can ask if the patient's illness (or injury) is urgent. If not urgent, they can give an appointment. If the caller feels it is urgent or is unsure, the call should be transferred to a nurse for triage. Clerical staff should receive instruction on recognizing true medical emergencies, calls that should immediately be directed to emergency medical services (EMS) or clinical personnel, as outlined in Table 2-1.

When reception/scheduling staff provide information that may seem simple (eg, dosage information for acetaminophen), they can place a physician and patient at considerable risk. Consider an example of a mother calling to ask the correct dosage of acetaminophen to treat her newborn's fever, but the receptionist fails to ascertain that the newborn is 3 weeks old. Or the mother who calls to ask the correct dosage of acetaminophen for the 18-month-old described earlier who has a low-grade fever, yet the receptionist does not ascertain that the child has petechiae as well. In these 2 examples, the caller is asking for simple information, but the patient has a potentially very serious illness that requires an urgent response. These calls require triage in addition to just providing simple answers to questions.

Table 2-1
Recognizing Emergent Calls

- Difficulty breathing (choking, stopped breathing, weak breathing, stridor, blue)

- Possible anaphylaxis (difficulty breathing or swallowing following medicine, bee stings, eating)

- Neurologic symptoms (seizure, loss of consciousness, hard to awaken, confusion)

- Poisoning, ingestion, or drug overdose

- Trauma to the neck or eye

- Uncontrollable bleeding

- Suicide threats or attempts and rape/abuse calls

- Fever in an infant younger than 3 months

- Fever greater than 104.5°F

- Inconsolable crying

- Chest pain

- Severe pain

- Near drowning

- Penetrating wounds

- Very anxious patient or caller

- Head trauma with behavior change or recurrent vomiting

- Purple or blood-colored rash

Trained clinical staff can triage the urgency of appointment requests. Callers insisting on an appointment or speaking to a physician should have their request reasonably met. If clinical staff or a physician cannot provide immediate advice, callers should be notified of when they might expect a return call and instructed to call back if the patient's condition worsens.

Telephone Care Providers Should Be Trained and Evaluated

Some offices choose to have an MA provide telephone care; others choose a licensed practical nurse or registered nurse. These decisions are highly influenced by the availability of applicants or by practice finances. *Physicians are accountable for advice given by any employee.* So telephone care should be delegated to the most experienced, best-trained person that the practice can find and afford. Telephone care providers represent the physician. They should function only under the direct supervision of a physician and must adhere to the scope of practice as defined by their licensure. Jurors expect whoever provides telephone care to be adequately trained and to have their performance regularly evaluated. When a nonphysician is found guilty of negligence or malpractice for telephone care, it usually has been the result of not documenting the call, not following available guidelines, or not consulting a physician.

The following strategies for reducing medicolegal risk for nonphysicians are recommended in the literature:

- Require the use of standardized telephone triage and advice guidelines for all clinical calls (Chapter 3).
- Establish an organized system for documenting all calls (Chapter 4).
- Provide and document training for the telephone care providers (Chapter 6).
- Regularly evaluate performance by observing calls and reviewing documentation (Chapter 7).
- Establish job descriptions that define the duties and limitations of the telephone care provider's role (Chapter 8).
- Establish dated policies and procedures (eg, addressing how to handle problem calls, caller discomfort, caller disagreement) (Chapter 9).
- Establish a quality improvement system for telephone care (Chapter 14).

Three additional, simple means for telephone care providers to reduce telephone liability include

- Ask whether the caller has additional questions or concerns.
- Ask whether the caller is comfortable with the advice and disposition and is able and willing to follow them.
- Advise the caller to call back if condition worsens or persists and provide specific things to watch for that would indicate the need to call back.

Malpractice Claims Are Lowest in Practices in Which the Physician Is Perceived as Accessible

The physician's schedule should accommodate all calls that the caller feels are urgent. Some of the highest-risk calls for a physician are those concerning true emergencies or when the caller perceives an urgent or emergent issue. Policies that do not allow staff to interrupt physicians with urgent phone calls during patient visits place the physician at increased risk. Likewise, physicians or their physician designees should be available 24 hours a day for potential urgent calls. Physicians who instruct the answering service to hold all calls while they attend a play or go out to dinner put themselves at increased medicolegal risk.

Judiciously and Reluctantly Prescribe Medications Over the Telephone in Keeping With State Law

Prescribing medication without seeing a patient obviously places a physician at risk. The risk is even greater when nonphysicians prescribe over the phone. Although most medications are well tolerated, side effects and allergic reactions do occur and can even cause serious harm to patients. When you prescribe over the phone, be sure to document what was prescribed, the dosage, follow-up instructions, and any discussion of side effects.

A Caller's Request to Have a Patient Seen Should Be Reasonably Met

A caller's request to have a patient seen should only reluctantly and carefully be denied, and the call should go through the complete triage process, using standardized telephone care guidelines. Callers may not be able to adequately convey in words their true concerns or the actual medical condition of the patient. Even if a thorough telephone assessment does not deem a face-to-face encounter necessary, respect a caller's concerns and honor his or her insistence that a patient be seen.

Do Not End Calls Until the Caller Understands and Agrees With the Plan

Bringing proper and complete closure to phone calls ensures that both parties have a mutual understanding of the situation and agree on a plan. Make it a habit to end each telephone call keeping in mind the 3 keys to a successful, low-risk closure.

1. Always clarify and repeat your assessment of the patient's condition.
2. Make sure the caller understands your instructions, including under what circumstances to call back.
3. Confirm that the caller is able and intends to comply with the plan. If a caller cannot, or does not, agree to comply with a plan and you are unable to meet the caller's needs, it is essential to document it.

Maintain Confidentiality

When the caller asks for information about a patient, always be careful to determine who is calling (and that it sounds believable to you). Determine to the best of your ability over the phone that the person has a legal right to ask for information about a patient. If the caller is a relative, an insurance company, or an estranged family member, ask about their relationship with the patient, where the patient is now, and whether the caller has a direct caregiving role or legal guardianship. When the person calling is not the patient, but the patient is available and a competent adult, ask to speak to the patient directly.

Provide Prompt, Courteous Service

Patients should have rapid access (within reason) to the office staff and physician. Office staff should monitor hold time (time callers spend on hold) and abandonment rates (number of callers on hold who hang up before the call can be answered), especially during peak calling times. If a menu-type voice recording (automated attendant) is used for initial call answering, callers should always first be instructed that if a potentially life-threatening emergency exists, they should hang up and call EMS (911). If it is necessary to place callers on hold, always ask first if they *can* hold for a moment.

If inbound clinical calls are not addressed immediately, physicians or their representative should strive to return calls as quickly as is reasonably possible. This reduces a physician's risk if the patient's condition worsens while waiting for a return call. Promptly returning calls also enhances patient satisfaction. Physicians should be familiar with the community standard for callback time during and after office hours.

After-Hours Telephone Care

A patient telephone call received when the office is closed is a source of greater liability than office-hours calls because patients are not as readily seen after hours and therefore may require a more sophisticated level of triage. It is generally assumed that primary care physicians are responsible for the medical care of their patients 24 hours a day (this is dictated by insurers and general public expectations). Physicians have a choice in how they wish to provide patients access to medical triage and advice after hours. Some physicians choose to use a recording that instructs callers with after-hours medical concerns to be seen at the nearest open medical facility. Most physicians avail themselves, a designated colleague, a nurse representative, or a combination to their patients for medical advice. The principles outlined previously for office-hours telephone calls apply to after-hours calls. However, some unique aspects of after-hours calls include the use of an answering service and, for some physicians, a nurse triage service.

Physicians choosing to provide after-hours advice generally use either an answering service or a telephone recording-type system with access to the physician by page. In either case, it should be clear to callers that if they have a perceived life-threatening emergency, they should immediately contact EMS. For all other calls, a message is usually left either on a recording or with an answering service. Callers should be informed how long it may take for their call to be returned and instructed to call again or to seek immediate medical care if the patient's condition worsens and becomes serious. Answering services are not qualified and should not be expected to triage the urgency of patient calls. An on-call physician should be paged for any caller requesting it.

The time it takes for a physician or his or her nurse representative to return an after-hours call varies greatly by region of the country and individual practices. It is recommended that physicians know their region's accepted callback time and adhere to it. For example, in Colorado, callback time for a nonurgent call during office hours is 1 to 2 hours and after hours is 30 to 60 minutes. Physicians who take longer than the standard time to return patient calls increase their risk if a patient's condition or outcome changes as a result of a delay in treatment.

Some family practices are now using after-hours nurse triage services. These services are well accepted by patients and physicians, and some medical malpractice carriers have lowered premiums for physicians using such services. Physicians should consider using these services as part of a risk-management program. To ensure that the nurse triage service provides quality service that may reduce risk, consider the program's qualifications as outlined in Chapter 21. Most importantly, even when after-hours care is delegated to a medical call center, primary care physicians share responsibility for all triage and advice provided to their patients. Juries have expected physicians to carefully review and select triage services and the guidelines they use. Telephone care guidelines used by nurses should be specific to the practice needs (eg, obstetrics, pediatrics, adult medicine) and up-to-date. Physicians also should make themselves readily available to the nurses and their patients for consultation.

Medicolegal Issues Associated With Managed Care

In addition to the already substantial liability associated with telephone care in general, managed care adds the additional risk associated with its objectives to limit access to care and direct patients to lower-cost providers and facilities. A backlash has formed in response to what the public perceives as limitation of care. Juries clearly have shown their disapproval of attempts to use the telephone to cut costs if there is a bad outcome. Most states have instituted new regulations requiring health plans to pay for emergency or urgent care for any condition that could be perceived by a reasonable layperson to be an urgent medical need, even if the primary care provider does not perceive the need to be urgent. It is acceptable, under these regulations, to make recommendations to callers about self-care or selection of site of care; but physicians in these states now have less authority to manage care by telephone, even though health plans provide incentives to do so. Therefore, telephone triage must be relatively conservative at the present time and should focus on quality care, patient satisfaction, and then appropriate resource use.

Conclusion

Telephone calls are considered a physician-patient encounter, and physicians are therefore legally responsible for medical advice given by themselves and their staff. Physicians can manage the risk associated with patient telephone calls through using careful call processing, delegating to qualified clinical staff, using standardized telephone care guidelines, and using standard, consistent documentation.

Chapter 3

Telephone Triage and Advice Guidelines

Although there are many important elements in a telephone care system, perhaps the single most important element to ensure quality and consistency and to reduce risk is the use of standardized telephone care guidelines. Telephone care guidelines assist telephone care providers through the interview, data collection, decision making, disposition selection, and advice-giving processes. The use of guidelines is recommended by the only accreditation agency for medical call centers, the American Accreditation Health Care Commission (formerly the Utilization Review Accreditation Commission). Clinical guidelines can now be found throughout the health care system. Their use is encouraged by medical societies, government agencies, managed care organizations, and risk-management groups.

Guideline Purpose and Goals

The use of telephone guidelines increases the likelihood that a group of telephone care providers will provide a standardized approach to care and decreases the likelihood of wide variations in care, some of which could be harmful. Even in offices where there is little triage and most ill patients are brought in for an office visit, the guidelines ensure that the home care advice provided by telephone is consistent from one nurse to another. Guidelines also improve nurses' productivity when dealing with unfamiliar symptoms. They simplify nurse training, expand nurse education, and provide a focus for physician review of nurse performance.

Determining the acuity or urgency of a patient's illness is not part of basic nursing training. Unlike physicians, most nurses have not seen the full range of serious complications that can be part of each acute illness. Moreover, in many states, the Nurse Practice Act requires that nurses use standardized guidelines if their role crosses over into medical practice, which can occur in providing telephone care.

Limitations

Triage guidelines do have limitations. They are a decision support tool, not a rigid protocol that should be strictly adhered to. They cannot tell a triager which guideline to use in a clinical situation, but they can offer options and assist with appropriate guideline selection. While they do not make diagnoses, they do help the triager determine the level of urgency of the patient's symptoms. Mainly they help the triager arrive at a safe and appropriate disposition, but only if they are used by a telephone care provider who is fully trained and capable of applying clinical judgment.

Experienced nurses using guidelines and clinical judgment on average override the guideline dispositions on 2% to 4% of calls. Usually the reasons include nurse discomfort with the patient's condition, the presence of an underlying chronic disease, or difficulty obtaining an adequate history from the caller. Some, but not all, of the variables can be built into the guidelines.

Selecting the Best Guideline for Each Call

The most difficult and important step in the entire process of using guidelines for telephone care is selecting the most appropriate guideline. It is not always obvious to the telephone care provider. Consult the description of how to select the best telephone care guideline provided in the guideline book that you purchase. The following are considerations to assist in this process:

- If the patient has one predominant symptom, use the guideline for that symptom.
- If there are multiple symptoms, select the most severe symptom or the one that appears to be the most emergent.
- If it is not clear which symptom is most severe or emergent, check the rank order of symptoms in the guideline book.
- Many guideline books suggest alternative guidelines to consider. Be sure to look at the alternative guidelines if you are unsure.
- For fever, use the guideline for the most serious associated symptom, unless fever is the only symptom.

Guideline Structure and Format

Guidelines generally can be organized into the following 7 components: symptom definition, selecting the most appropriate guideline, initial assessment questions, telephone triage questions, first-aid advice, telephone care advice, and callback advice. Examples of headache guidelines are found in tables 3-1 and 3-2.

Symptom Definition

Most guidelines are symptom based. Often symptoms mentioned by the patient can be accepted at face value (eg, earache, cough, head injury, nosebleed), but sometimes the definition requires some clarification. For example, an infant's normal spitting up and reflux must be differentiated from vomiting. Nurses should ensure that the caller's definition is the same as the guideline definition for the symptom of concern.

In general, neither the patient nor the triage nurse makes diagnoses. However, there are many illnesses that patients can recognize (eg, the common cold, athlete's foot, head lice). Patients may have had other family members diagnosed with the same disease or have friends or neighbors who suggest the diagnosis to them. For these, a disease-based guideline (rather than a symptom-based guideline) may be warranted as long as the caller's description of the symptoms complies with the diagnostic criteria for the guideline. The most quoted serious error in accepting a patient's diagnosis over the telephone is a child who has a petechial rash with meningococcemia the parent mistakenly believes is chickenpox.

Selecting the Most Appropriate Guideline

Each guideline book should provide direction on how to find the most appropriate guideline for each call. Often the guideline itself will have prompts to help the triage nurse select the most appropriate guideline. The nurse can use these prompts to rethink the caller's main concern. Symptom-based guidelines may redirect the triager to a more specific disease-based guideline (eg, from Cough to Asthma). If asthma is causing the cough, more targeted triage and advice will be found in the asthma guideline. For disease-based guidelines, if the

---

Table 3-1
Headache Guideline for Children

Symptom Definition
- Pain or discomfort of the scalp or forehead areas
- The face and ears are excluded.

Causes
- The main causes are muscle tension headaches and headaches from fever.
- Sudden-onset headaches that are excruciating and incapacitating are usually migraines.

See Other Protocol
- TRAUMA, HEAD

Initial Assessment Questions
1. LOCATION: "Where does it hurt?"
2. DURATION: "When did the headache start?" (Minutes, hours, or days)
3. CONSTANT OR INTERMITTENT: "Does the pain come and go, or has it been constant since it started?"
   (Note: serious pain is constant and usually worsens)
4. SEVERITY: "How bad is the pain?" and "What does it keep your child from doing?"
   – Mild: interferes minimally or not at all with activities
   – Moderate: interferes with normal activities or awakens from sleep
   – Severe: excruciating pain and child screaming or incapacitated
5. RECURRENT SYMPTOM: "Has your child ever had headaches before?" If so, ask: "When was the last time?"
   and "what happened that time?"
6. CAUSE: "What do you think is causing the headache?"
7. HEAD INJURY: "Has there been any recent injury to the head?"
8. MIGRAINE: "Is there any family history for migraine headaches?"
9. CHILD'S APPEARANCE: "How does your child look?" "What is he doing right now?"

TRIAGE ASSESSMENT QUESTIONS FOR HEADACHE

Activate Emergency Medical Services (911)
- Difficult to awaken   (R/O increased intracranial pressure)

See Immediately in Emergency Department or Office (ask primary care physician)
- Neurological symptoms   (R/O encephalitis, subdural hematoma)
   – Confused thinking   – Blurred or double vision   – Slurred speech
   – Unsteady walking   – Weakness
- Stiff neck   (R/O meningitis, subarachnoid bleed)
- Child sounds very sick or weak to the triager   (R/O serious cause)

See Immediately in Office
- Severe headache with fever   (R/O sinusitis, meningitis)
- Vomited 2 or more times (EXCEPTION: previous migraine headaches)
       (R/O ICP, strep pharyngitis, first migraine)
- Fever >105°F (40.6°C) rectally or orally   (R/O serious bacterial infection)

(continued on page 16)

<table>
<tr><td>

Table 3-1
Headache Guideline for Children, continued

</td></tr>
<tr><td>

See Today
- Parent wants child seen
- Sore throat present >24 hours (R/O strep throat)
- Sinus pain or pressure of forehead (R/O frontal sinusitis)
- Severe headache not improved with pain medicine (R/O first migraine)
- Headache present >24 hours (R/O sinusitis or other treatable cause)
  (EXCEPTION: analgesics not yet tried, or headache is part of a generalized illness)

See Within 2 Weeks
- Recurrent headaches (R/O tension headaches, migraine, school avoidance)

Home Care
- Mild headache

HOME CARE ADVICE FOR MILD HEADACHES

1. **Reassure the Caller:** It doesn't sound like a serious headache.

2. **Pain Medicine:** Give acetaminophen or ibuprofen for pain relief. (See dosage tables in Appendix.)
   Headaches due to fever are also helped by fever reduction.

3. **Food:** Give fruit juice or food if your child is hungry or hasn't eaten in >4 hours.
   (Reason: Skipping a meal can cause a headache in many children.)

4. **Rest:** Lie down in a quiet place and relax until feeling better.

5. **Local Cold:** Apply a cold, wet washcloth or cold pack to the forehead for 20 minutes.

6. **Stretching:** Stretch and massage any tight neck muscles.

7. **Call back if**
- Severe headache persists >2 hours after pain medicine
- Headache lasts >24 hours despite using a pain medicine

Resources
Elser JM. Easing the pain of childhood headaches. *Contemp Pediatr.* 1991;8:108–123
Feigin RD, McCracken GH Jr, Klein JO. Diagnosis and management of meningitis. *Pediatr Infect Dis J.* 1992;11:785–814
Forsyth R, Farrell K. Headache in childhood. *Pediatr Rev.* 1999;20:39–45
Molofsky WJ. Headaches in children. *Pediatr Ann.* 1998;27:614–621

</td></tr>
</table>

Adapted from Schmitt BD. *Pediatric Telephone Protocols: Office Version.* 9th ed. Elk Grove Village, IL: American Academy of Pediatrics; 2002.

diagnostic criteria are not met, the triage nurse can be redirected to the appropriate symptom guideline (eg, from Hives to Rash, Widespread and Cause Unknown).

Initial Assessment Questions

The initial assessment questions associated with each symptom or disease help the triage nurse capture a snapshot of the patient's present condition. They help the nurse better define the symptoms and their duration. They also document how much the patient's symptoms

Table 3-2
Headache Guideline for Adults

Symptom Definition
- Pain or discomfort of the scalp or forehead areas
- The face and ears are excluded

Background Information
Common Causes
- During the course of a year, the majority of adults suffer headaches.
- **Muscle Tension Headaches:** The majority of headaches are caused by muscle tension. The discomfort is usually diffuse and may radiate down into the neck and shoulders. The discomfort is aggravated by emotional stress.
- **Migraine Headaches:** Also referred to as vascular headaches. The headache is moderate to severe in intensity, described as throbbing or pulsing in nature, and usually unilateral. Associated symptoms include nausea and vomiting. Some individuals will have visual warning symptoms (aura) that a migraine is coming.
- **Sinusitis:** Headaches occur with sinusitis. The headache is usually located in the forehead area and the individual has associated sinus symptoms (nasal discharge, congestion).
- **Fever:** A mild to moderate headache frequently accompanies the fever that occurs with common viral infections such as the flu and the common cold. A severe headache that persists after the fever has come down to normal is a red flag that something more serious may be causing the headache.
- **Caffeine Withdrawal:** This occurs in individuals who drink large amounts of caffeine (eg, coffee, tea, colas) and suddenly stop. Some caffeine drinkers will note a headache upon arising that goes away after their first cup of coffee.

See Other Protocol
- TRAUMA, HEAD
- SINUS PAIN AND CONGESTION

TRIAGE ASSESSMENT QUESTIONS FOR HEADACHE

Call EMS 911 NOW
- Difficult to awaken or acting confused (disoriented, slurred speech)   R/O: subarachnoid hemorrhage, meningitis
- Weakness of the face, arm, or leg on one side of the body (new onset)   R/O: stroke
- Numbness of the face, arm, or leg on one side of the body (new onset)
- Loss of speech or garbled speech (new onset)
- Passed out
- Sounds like a life-threatening emergency to the triager

See NOW in ED (or Office With PCP Approval)
- Unsteady walking   R/O: encephalitis
- Stiff neck (cannot touch chin to chest)   R/O: meningitis
- Severe pain in one eye   R/O: angle-closure glaucoma
- Possibility of carbon monoxide exposure   R/O: CO poisoning
- Severe pain, states "worst headache" of life   R/O: migraine, CNS bleed
- Patient sounds very sick or weak to the triager

Table 3-2
Headache Guideline for Adults, continued

See NOW in Office
- Pain is severe and has not had severe headaches before — R/O: new-onset migraine, CNS bleed, brain tumor
- Fever >103°F (39.4°C) — R/O: bacterial infection
- Fever >100.5°F (38.1°C) and diabetes mellitus or immunocompromised (eg, HIV positive, cancer chemotherapy, chronic steroid treatment) — R/O: meningitis, encephalitis
- Blurred vision — R/O: temporal arteritis

Callback by PCP or Subspecialist
- Pain is severe and has had severe headaches before — R/O: migraine
- Vomiting — R/O: migraine, increased ICP

See Today in Office
- Patient wants to be seen
- Severe sore throat — R/O: pharyngitis
- New headache and age >50 — Reason: greater risk of organic pathology
- New headache and immunocompromised (eg, HIV positive, cancer chemotherapy, chronic steroid treatment)
- Sinus pain or pressure of forehead and nasal symptoms (discharge) — R/O: frontal sinusitis
- Fever present >3 days — R/O: sinusitis
- Unexplained headache that is present >24 hours — R/O: sinusitis or other treatable cause

See Within 2 Weeks in the Office
- Headaches are a recurrent, ongoing problem — R/O: tension headaches, migraine headaches

Home Care
- Mild-moderate headache — R/O: tension headache
- Headache similar to prior migraines — R/O: migraine headache

HOME CARE ADVICE FOR HEADACHE

1. **Pain Medication:** For pain relief, take acetaminophen every 4-6 hours (adult dosage 650 mg) OR ibuprofen every 6-8 hours (adult dosage 400 mg).
   - Do not take ibuprofen if you have stomach problems, kidney disease, are pregnant, or have been told by your doctor to avoid this type of anti-inflammatory drug. Do not take ibuprofen for more than 7 days without consulting your doctor.
   - Do not take acetaminophen if you have liver disease.
   - Read the package instructions thoroughly on all medications that you take.

2. **Migraine Medication:** If your doctor has prescribed specific medication for your migraine, take it as directed as soon as the migraine starts.

Table 3-2
Headache Guideline for Adults, continued

3. **Rest:**
   - Lie down in a dark quiet place and try to relax. Close your eyes and imagine your entire body relaxing.
   - Try to fall asleep. Individuals with migraines often awaken from sleep with their headache relieved.

4. **Local Cold:** Apply a cold wet washcloth or cold pack to the forehead for 20 minutes.

5. **Stretching:** Stretch and massage any tight neck muscles.

6. **Call Back If:**
   - Severe headache
   - Headache last longer than 24 hours
   - You become worse.

Some Serious Causes of Headache
- Stroke ("Brain Attack")
- Meningitis, encephalitis
- Temporal arteritis
- Brain tumor
- Carbon monoxide exposure

References and Resources
Newman LC, Lipton RB. Emergency department evaluation of headache. *Neurol Clin*. 1998;16:285–303
Saper JR. Medicolegal issues: headache. *Neurol Clin*. 1999;17:197–214
Sheftell FD. Role and impact of over-the-counter medications in the management of headache. *Neurol Clin*. 1997;15:187–198
Silberstein SD. Drug-induced headache. *Neurol Clin*. 1998;16:107–123
Sztajnkrycer M, Jauch EC. Unusual headaches. *Emerg Med Clin North Am*. 1998;16:741–760, vi

Reviewed and Authorized by: _____

Adapted from Thompson DA. *Adult Telephone Triage Protocols: Office Version*. Elk Grove Village, IL: American Academy of Pediatrics. In press.

interfere with normal daily activities. These general questions should be asked before moving on to the triage questions, which explore possible complications of the illness.

Telephone Triage Questions

In most telephone care guidelines, triage questions are listed in a logical sequence from most severe to least severe etiologies for that symptom. Questions are designed to include a differential diagnosis for that symptom. The triage questions must be asked in order, from conditions of highest to lowest acuity (most serious to least serious diagnoses). If an answer is negative, one moves on to the next question. A positive answer to a triage question categorizes a patient into a particular disposition or action and further questioning stops.

Triage Disposition Categories

Selecting a useful time frame of disposition categories is the heart of all telephone care guideline systems. Triage guidelines determine which patients need to be seen rather than cared for at home. They also determine when and where the patient needs to be seen. Triage guidelines try to strike a balance between under-referral and over-referral. Under-referral can lead to delayed visits, delayed diagnosis, delayed treatment, and serious complications. Examples would be not bringing in to evaluate a patient with appendicitis, foreign body aspiration, or meningitis. Over-referral risks mainly apply to after-hours care and unnecessary emergency department (ED) visits. During office hours, over-referral has negative consequences for the physician and patient if it is an unnecessary use of time, particularly for the working patient, leading to loss of work time and possibly of wages.

Telephone triage must be based on a spectrum of disposition categories ranging from activating emergency medical services (EMS) for life-threatening emergencies to not seeing the patient at all (caring for the patient at home because the illness or injury is mild). Dispositions useful for an office system are listed in Table 3-3. They are based on a survey that

Table 3-3 **Triage Disposition Categories or Time Frames**
Activate emergency medical services (911) immediately (life-threatening emergencies).
See immediately (emergent patients). – Office. – Emergency department. – Discuss site with primary care physician.
See today by appointment (urgent or uncomfortable patients).
See today or tomorrow by appointment (nonurgent patients).
See within 2 weeks (recurrent or persistent symptoms).
Do not see and home care (mildly ill patients).

Table 3-4 Distribution of Office-Hours Calls by Disposition	
Activate emergency medical services (911)	<1%
See immediately in emergency department	1%
See immediately in office	2% - 9%
See today or tomorrow in office	50% - 60%
Home care	30% - 40%

asked 100 Denver, CO, primary care physicians how they would refer urgent or emergent symptoms. The Activate EMS (911) disposition should contain questions that detect life-threatening emergencies. The See Immediately disposition should contain questions that help to detect patients with potential emergent or urgent conditions who should be seen within 2 hours. The See Within 24 Hours by Appointment disposition should contain the questions required to identify the remaining patients who should be seen today or tomorrow and cannot safely be managed at home. When the office is open, most patients who need to be seen are given a same-day appointment. The Home Care disposition identifies those patients whose medical condition can be safely managed at home.

Table 3-4 lists the percentage of patients who fall within each disposition category based on an average day's calls. The percentage of patients cared for at home without an office visit will increase if the office provides more telephone triage and advice. It also increases if patients are encouraged to consult with the advice nurse before requesting an appointment.

First-Aid Advice

If the patient has a life-threatening or serious emergency, first-aid instructions should be provided. The purpose of first aid is to minimize injury and damage before the patient is transported to the ED or office. Examples range from giving an adrenaline injection for possible anaphylactic reaction to applying cold water to an acute burn.

Telephone Care Advice

This section of the guideline contains home treatment advice that should be offered to any patient who does not need to be seen immediately or who does not need a health care visit. For specific diseases, the advice should be in keeping with standard textbooks of family medicine. For symptoms, advice usually is given for treating the 1 or 2 most common causes of that symptom. Nonprescription medications may be mentioned (eg, antihistamines) with appropriate dosages. The expected course of the symptom or disease should be provided so that patients will know what to expect. For infectious diseases, it is helpful to include information about the contagious period and incubation period. If the condition has a strong propensity to recur, preventive advice should be given.

Callback Advice

Every call should end with callback instructions (contingency plan). This should include a list of the 2 or 3 most likely complications plus the generic statements "if you become worse" or "if you are concerned." If any of them occur, the caller should know to call the office again.

Selection of a Guideline Book

The selection of a book of telephone care guidelines should follow a logical process. First, review the existing books that contain telephone guidelines. (See Bibliography.) Then compare the management of 3 common symptoms in each of the books. Have a checklist of your requirements.

- The number of symptoms covered is comprehensive (usually more than 100 topics).
- Directions for selecting the most appropriate guideline are included.
- The disposition categories are compatible with office practice options and scheduling.
- The decision-making process is easy to follow.
- Life-threatening emergencies are included, easily recognized, and dealt with quickly.
- The care advice is clear, easy to understand, and specific.
- Callback instructions are present and specific.
- The triage and advice is internally consistent from one guideline to the next.
- The content is up-to-date and referenced to the current literature.
- The content has undergone a review process.
- The content has been widely used or tested in office settings.

Review Process for Guidelines

Much of the content of telephone guidelines cannot be supported by existing research. However, content can be linked to the current standard of practice and supported by expert review. Reviewers should include practicing family physicians. Selected specialized guidelines should be reviewed by subspecialists and surgeons. You should verify that the guidelines you intend to purchase have been reviewed prior to publication.

A physician in your practice should review the guidelines completely prior to implementing them in your practice. The factors that should be considered in your review process follow.

Implementing Preexisting Guidelines in Office Practice

The advantages of purchasing preexisting guidelines are many. They are already completed and available, and they have already undergone a review process and testing in other offices. The referral rates for different dispositions are already known. And most importantly, they save the tremendous resources and time needed to create original guidelines (it is estimated that it requires an average of 10-12 hours to complete 1 guideline). Using guidelines with an established standard of care avoids protracted discussions among participating physicians related to normal variations in practice patterns. Overall, the most cost-effective approach is to buy and implement an existing telephone guideline book.

If existing telephone guidelines are used, they can be customized to suit practice-specific needs. In general, any changes should be standardized for all members of the group to decrease confusion for the triage nurse. Customizing the guidelines differently for each practitioner decreases the ability of the nurse to memorize standard advice and also adversely affects productivity. There are few reasons to modify the triage questions. When practices modify telephone care guidelines it is usually to either (1) make changes in home care advice, recommended over-the-counter medications, and indicate which prescriptions can be called in or (2) adapt the disposition sites (office or ED) recommended for specific emergent conditions.

To customize existing guidelines, any sentence or paragraph the practitioner disagrees with can be crossed out. To replace a paragraph, the new version can be typed and taped over the existing one. To add additional advice, the additional instructions can be typed and taped at the end of the guideline to which it applies. It is important for medicolegal purposes that all changes be documented (reflecting the original and new language), dated, and signed for approval.

Before launching a new telephone advice system, nurses should be trained. This is best accomplished by having them study the guidelines themselves, starting with the 10 or 20 most common calls. Keep in mind that the 10 most common symptoms cover 50% of calls and the top 25 cover 80%. (Table 3-5 ranks the top 25 symptoms.) Selecting the most appropriate guideline may be the most difficult part of the nurse's assignment. The guideline materials that you select should have tips for choosing the most appropriate guidelines in specific cases. Most will include prompts that help providers work through the options. Most importantly, the triager needs to know that if the patient seems very sick, based on initial assessment questions, he or she should be seen immediately, even if no indicator is met within the guideline. Many guideline manuals are accompanied by a user's manual that can be read by the nurse before taking any calls. For full information on training, see Chapter 6.

Customizing Dispositions for Potential Emergencies

After life-threatening emergencies have been referred to EMS (911), patients with potential emergencies usually receive better care if they first come to the office. If the patient might need referral to a specialist, it makes more sense for the primary care physician to provide this initial assessment than for the patient to make an extra stop in the ED. The primary care physician can see the patient faster. The office setting is less stressful for the patient. The primary care physician usually needs less laboratory work and fewer imaging studies to reach a decision than does an ED physician. The primary care physician can evaluate the patient in the most cost-effective manner.

These comments also are based on the fact that most offices do provide many urgent procedures, including nebulizer treatments, suturing, minor burn care, wound and bite irrigation, and basic laboratory tests. Another factor to consider is the accuracy of patient reporting over the telephone. Most patients cannot accurately assess dehydration, difficulty in breathing, stiff neck, and other potentially serious symptoms. Referral of all patients who are suspected of having these conditions after a telephone assessment could lead to unnecessary visits to the ED.

Because of wide variation in the comfort level of practicing physicians for evaluation of potentially emergent symptoms, telephone care guidelines for office practice may suggest asking the primary care physician to decide whether patients with such symptoms can best be cared for in the office or referred directly to a surgeon or subspecialist or to the ED. The

Table 3-5
Pediatric Calls: The Top 25 Symptoms
1. Upper respiratory illness
2. Fever
3. Earache
4. Abdominal pain
5. Vomiting, nausea
6. Diarrhea
7. Sore throat, swollen glands
8. Backache
9. Headache
10. Minor trauma of the extremity
11. Rash
12. Eye infection
13. High blood pressure
14. Chest pain
15. Dysuria, frequency
16. Dizziness
17. Difficulty breathing
18. Joint pain
19. Asthma
20. Fatigue
21. Laceration
22. Lumps, masses
23. Complications from diabetes
24. Anxiety
25. Side effect from medication

Adapted from Fischer PM, Smith SR. The nature and management of telephone utilization in a family practice setting. *J Fam Pract.* 1979;8:321–327 and Spencer DC, Daugird AJ. The nature and content of physician telephone calls in a private practice. *J Fam Pract.* 1988;27:201–205.

physician can speak directly to the caller or make a decision based on information from the triage nurse.

Keeping Guidelines Current

All clinical guidelines should be reviewed and updated on a yearly basis by a physician in the practice. First and foremost, they should be kept consistent with current medical literature. Examples include listing the side effects of new vaccines, adding new standards from national guidelines on disease management (eg, National Institutes of Health guidelines on home management of asthma), or adding new precautions (eg, avoiding ibuprofen in children with chickenpox because of the potential increased risk of invasive strep infections). A second source of updates is the informal feedback from triage nurse users. A third source is the formal evaluation as part of quality improvement (QI) programs performed within large offices or call centers. (See Chapter 14.) A final source of new information is published research and outcome studies.

Written Versus Computerized Guidelines

Most offices will function most efficiently using written guidelines. A large multispecialty group (usually more than 50 physicians) with centralized triage services may elect to have its guidelines become computerized, especially if the group already has electronic medical records. Some advantages of computerized guidelines include

- Registration: Previous callers are preregistered.
- Health history: Patients with chronic diseases are flagged. The availability of medical histories reduces the risk of overlooking chronic disease complications and allows for more personalized calls.
- Care advice: Targeted care advice can be provided for each triage question in the software version.
- Documentation: The documentation of each call is more comprehensive with software. Data retrieval also is easier from software than from filing cabinets of hard copies.
- Risk management: Software encourages better compliance with the triage guidelines by the triage nurse. Also, having all calls automatically documented and stored electronically reduces medical liability.
- Total quality management program: quality assessment and QI objectives are easier to achieve using computerized data.

Disadvantages of computerized guidelines include

- Increased cost: Not only is there the increased cost of the software, but the added cost of hardware. Printed guidelines are relatively inexpensive.
- Increased skills: Triage nurses need keyboarding and computer skills.
- Longer calls: Call times are usually 1 or 2 minutes longer.
- Duplication: Intermittent computer system shutdowns require duplicate written guidelines for backup use.

Summary

Clinical guidelines have standardized the process of telephone data collection, decision making, and advice giving. The critical element of a guideline system is a disposition timetable that matches the service options available in office practice. Guidelines also should be compatible with the current literature and American Academy of Family Physicians policy statements. They need to undergo a formal review process and be updated on a regular basis. When office nurses provide telephone triage and advice, adherence to clinical guidelines has become the standard of care.

Bibliography

Telephone Care Books/Guidelines

General Guidelines

Briggs JK. *Telephone Triage Protocols for Nurses.* 2nd ed. Philadelphia, PA: Lippincott Williams & Wilkins; 2002

Brown JL. *Pediatric Telephone Medicine: Principles, Triage, and Advice.* 2nd ed. Philadelphia, PA: Lippincott Williams & Wilkins; 1994

Katz HP. *Telephone Medicine: Triage and Training for Primary Care.* 2nd ed. Philadelphia, PA: F. A. Davis Co; 2001

Pediatric Guidelines

Schmitt BD. *Pediatric Telephone Protocols: After-Hours Version.* 9th ed. Littleton, CO: Decision Press; 2002

Schmitt BD. *Pediatric Telephone Protocols: Office Version.* 9th ed. Elk Grove Village, IL: American Academy of Pediatrics; 2002

Wheeler SQ. *Telephone Triage Protocols for Infants and Children: Birth to 6 Years.* Gaithersburg, MD: Aspen Publishers; 1997

Adult Guidelines

Thompson DA. *Adult Telephone Protocols: Office Version.* Elk Grove Village, IL: American Academy of Pediatrics; 2004

Wheeler SQ. *Telephone Triage Protocols for Adults 18 Years and Older.* Gaithersburg, MD: Aspen Publishers; 1997

Obstetric-Gynecologic Guidelines

Long VE, McMullen PC. *Telephone Triage for Obstetrics and Gynecology.* Philadelphia, PA: Lippincott Williams & Wilkins; 2002

Swenson DE. *Telephone Triage of the Obstetric Patient: A Nursing Guide.* 2nd ed. Philadelphia, PA: WB Saunders Co; 2001

Chapter 4

Documentation of Telephone Care

Even though your practice provides exemplary care, if there is a bad outcome you may be considered liable unless the proper care is adequately documented. Documentation is an important method of communicating among practice members about the clinical care provided by telephone, and it also enhances other office functions, such as medical record keeping, continuity of care, complaint resolution, patient care follow-up, and quality assurance. The most time-efficient method is to use telephone call documentation forms, which incorporate prompts to remind the provider what to document and checklists to make it quick and easy.

From a medicolegal standpoint, all calls during which a nonphysician provides triage, advice, or health information should be documented. Physician calls requiring documentation include those in which medical advice is given, a change in treatment is made, advice about a medication is given, a patient is directed to see a health care provider, a positive test is reported, or symptoms are potentially serious. Good documentation allows other members of the practice to have sufficient information about each patient encounter.

When telephone care guidelines are used, documentation can be expedited by indicating which guideline was used, briefly documenting the positive responses to questions from the guideline, and noting "advice per guideline." Minimal documentation for clinical calls should include the following information:

- Demographics: caller name, relationship to the patient and phone number, patient name and age (or date of birth), date and time of call
- Clinical information: reason for call or presenting complaint, main symptoms (no more than 1 or 2 sentences or phrases)
- Guideline(s) used and pertinent positives on the questions in the guideline(s)
- Disposition recommended by the guideline(s)
- Advice given (it is acceptable to write "per guideline"), medications suggested and dosages, and callback instructions (can write "per guideline")
- Caller understanding and acceptance of advice
- Signature of telephone care provider

For medicolegal purposes, paper documentation should be done in ink (not pencil). Documentation of clinical calls must be retrievable. Most practices will place telephone documentation in the chart. However, from a medicolegal standpoint, documentation of routine calls does not necessarily have to be in the chart. Such documentation can be retained in telephone call logs as long as it is retrievable. Calls that definitely should be in the chart include those relating to serious or chronic illness, clinical calls from another health professional, and those calls that require a physician's input.

Consider creating documentation forms or log books for your practice using carbon or no-carbon-required (NCR) paper to create at least 1 copy. Some practices prefer small third- or half-page forms to economize on space in the chart; other practices prefer full-page forms to have ample room to document.

The following are 3 sample documentation forms or log sheets that you may use or adapt for your practice:

Example of a Telephone Care Documentation Form for Office Hours		
Date: *5/21/98* **Time:** *0904* **Caller:** *Beth Dawson, Mom* **Patient:** *Dawson, Sue* **Phone:** *555-0201* **Age:** *11 years* **Gender:** M ☐ F ☑ **Nurse:** *J. Cameron* **Pharmacy:** *555-1111*	**Symptoms** *Runny nose x 2-3 weeks clear discharge, eyes itch* **Other info:** *Wt 82 lbs* **Allergies:** *none* **Meds:** *none* **Chronic disease:** *none* **Guideline used:** *Hay fever* **Advice:** *per guideline* **Meds:** *CTM 8 mg LA tab* **Dose:** *1 every 12 h* **Call back:** *if Sx not controlled on this med*	**Disposition** ☐ See immediately 　☐ Office ☐ ED ☐ 911 ☐ See today ☐ See tomorrow and 　protocol advice given ☐ Later appointment ☑ Home care advice per 　guideline ☑ Caller understands ☑ Caller agrees ☐ Refer call to MD ☐ Override reason:

This form adapted with permission from Schmitt BD. *Pediatric Telephone Protocols: Office Version*. 9th ed. Elk Grove Village, IL: American Academy of Pediatrics; 2002. Permission to photocopy granted.

Sample Telephone Log Sheet

TELEPHONE LOG SHEET

Triage Nurse _____

Date _____

Time	Phone #	Patient Age	Symptom or Problem	Chronic Disease	Protocol Used	Disposition	Advice Per Protocol	Drug Dose

From Schmitt BD. *Pediatric Telephone Protocols: Office Version.* 9th ed. Elk Grove Village, IL: American Academy of Pediatrics; 2002. Reprinted with permission. Permission to photocopy granted.

Sample Telephone Log Sheet		

Date
 	
Time
 	
Patient Name
 	
Age
 	
Sex: M ☐   F ☐
 	
Phone Number
 	
Nurse
	Symptoms:
	
	Protocol used _____ ☐
	
	Chronic disease _____
	
	Drug_____
	
	Dose _____
	
	Other info:
		☐ See immediately
		  ☐ Office ☐ ED ☐ 911
		☐ See today
		☐ See tomorrow and
		  protocol advice given
		
		☐ Later appointment
		☐ Home care and protocol
		  advice given
		
		☐ Caller agrees
		☐ Refer call to MD

Date
 	
Time
 	
Patient Name
 	
Age
 	
Sex: M ☐   F ☐
 	
Phone Number
 	
Nurse
	Symptoms:
	
	Protocol used _____ ☐
	
	Chronic disease _____
	
	Drug_____
	
	Dose _____
	
	Other info:
		☐ See immediately
		  ☐ Office ☐ ED ☐ 911
		☐ See today
		☐ See tomorrow and
		  protocol advice given
		
		☐ Later appointment
		☐ Home care and protocol
		  advice given
		
		☐ Caller agrees
		☐ Refer call to MD

Date
 	
Time
 	
Patient Name
 	
Age
 	
Sex: M ☐   F ☐
 	
Phone Number
 	
Nurse
	Symptoms:
	
	Protocol used _____ ☐
	
	Chronic disease _____
	
	Drug_____
	
	Dose _____
	
	Other info:
		☐ See immediately
		  ☐ Office ☐ ED ☐ 911
		☐ See today
		☐ See tomorrow and
		  protocol advice given
		
		☐ Later appointment
		☐ Home care and protocol
		  advice given
		
		☐ Caller agrees
		☐ Refer call to MD

From Schmitt BD. *Pediatric Telephone Protocols: Office Version.* 9th ed. Elk Grove Village, IL: American Academy of Pediatrics; 2002. Reprinted with permission. Permission to photocopy granted.

Chapter 5

Delegating Telephone Care to Nonphysicians and Selecting Telephone Care Staff

This chapter may be the most controversial one. Although there are insufficient outcome research data to assist you in making this important decision, you must determine what level of training for a telephone provider is adequate to promote quality telephone care and still be affordable for the practice. Almost as difficult is recognizing the qualities that are needed to become a skilled telephone care provider.

Delegating telephone care to nonphysicians improves call flow, patient flow in the office, physician satisfaction, documentation, and patient education. In addition, delegating telephone care to nonphysicians generally is well accepted by patients, with nearly all callers equally content to speak with a nurse, medical assistant, or physician. While many offices employ non-nurses to provide clinical care by telephone, medical call centers require that registered nurses (RNs) provide telephone triage and advice. This chapter provides the information you will require in selecting telephone care providers for your practice.

From studies of primary care practices, we know that practices vary greatly in terms of who provides telephone care. These studies have shown that options include physicians, mid-level practitioners, RNs, licensed practical nurses (LPNs), medical assistants (MAs), health assistants, and reception/scheduling (clerical) staff. Those primarily responsible for providing telephone care during office hours in the practices studied were RNs (36%), physicians (24%), LPNs (20%), MAs (18%), and reception/scheduling staff (14%). Physicians, while most qualified, are 4 to 6 times more expensive than nurses. Mid-level practitioners can handle 90% to 95% of calls, but are often twice as expensive as nurses. Registered nurses are the most expensive nursing option and the best prepared, as they usually have 4 years of training. Licensed practical nurses receive 2 years of training and are less expensive, but they require more physician supervision and involvement. Medical assistants have only 9 months of training. Health assistants are office staff with no clinical training or licensure. It is generally accepted that health assistants and reception/scheduling (clerical) staff should not provide telephone care.

Early studies and reports suggest that possessing nursing education and expertise improves the performance of someone who provides telephone triage and advice. In one study, decisions made by health assistants were compared to those made by nurses. The results indicated that health assistants made significantly more decisions that the physician did not agree with. In addition, nurses in the study were able to handle 15% more calls without needing physician input, compared to health assistants. It is important to note that those studies were done in an era before telephone care guidelines commonly were used. Today, use of guidelines is commonplace but, unfortunately, there are no studies that compare the performance of providers with different levels of training when all use telephone care guidelines.

It may be tempting to delegate telephone care to uncertified health assistants, or even to clerical staff with no formal training, as a way to reduce costs. This may be a false economy because such workers may require assistance from nurses or physicians on a higher proportion of calls. We recommend that practices select telephone care providers who have as much training and experience as the practices can afford. We also recommend that telephone care providers have considerable clinical experience, have telephone experience, be trained in telephone care, follow standardized clinical guidelines, completely document calls, and have physician backup. Because after-hours telephone care usually has less physician supervision and because more patients are triaged away from urgent care than during office hours, after-hours care should be delegated to a nurse rather than an MA or health assistant.

Selecting Telephone Care Staff

Once you have decided what level of health care training you want the telephone care provider in your practice to have, you will want to think about what other specific experience, characteristics, and criteria will help you identify people with the best aptitude to provide telephone care. Typically, nurses from an ambulatory setting or whose experience is in primary care find the transition to telephone care easier than nurses who come from highly specialized inpatient settings. While there are no perfect predictors of success, the following criteria often improve a person's aptitude for providing telephone care:

- Previous primary care office experience (at least 2 years), previous experience in an emergency department, or previous ambulatory care experience
- Good interpersonal and communication skills
- Experience in providing telephone care
- Ability to direct the flow of a telephone call and reach closure in an efficient manner
- Ability to do more than one thing at a time (multitasking)
- Good telephone "presence"
- Empathy and good listening skills
- Ability to work independently
- Common sense
- Problem-solving skills
- Ability to calculate medication dosages
- The ability to type at least 35 words per minute if documenting electronically

Because it is very important that telephone care providers present themselves well on the phone, it is wise to conduct at least a portion of the hiring interview over the phone to assess their telephone demeanor and skills. How well do they communicate in a non–face-to-face situation? Is their voice pleasant? Are they an efficient communicator? Can they "read" you over the phone? Do they listen carefully to the caller? Was the telephone portion of the interview taken seriously? When the call ended, were you pleased with the interaction? These same considerations also apply when you are hiring an answering service or after-hours telephone care call center.

Attracting Telephone Care Providers

In many areas of the country there is a nursing shortage, and recruiting experienced people may be difficult. It may be helpful to offer part-time positions, flexible hours, or a 9-months-per-year contract (to allow working parents to be at home during the summer with children). It is helpful to have a pleasant work space with attention to ergonomics. It also is helpful to have a special status for telephone care providers, manifested by a separate job description, compensation rate, and title. The topic of retention of staff is addressed in Chapter 17.

Chapter 6

Training Telephone Care Providers

This chapter provides the core training material and should be required reading for all members of the practice staff who provide telephone care. It also introduces a new concept, the model call, which will improve cost-efficiency more than any other element of the telephone care system. Defining the model call is a step that practices may be tempted to bypass; however, in addition to reducing cost, it also improves the efficiency of the training process and standardization of care.

Telephone care is one of the most difficult aspects of medical care.

- Communication is limited and nuances of face-to-face communication are absent.
- The provider usually obtains less information than during an office visit and has less time in which to make a decision.
- The provider cannot examine and usually does not talk to the patient.
- The provider often is not familiar with the patient.
- Patients are increasingly complex.
- The demand for telephone care is increasing.

Despite the fact that telephone care requires great skill and experience, the paucity of training for physicians and nurses in telephone care has been documented in many studies. Until recently, nursing schools have not included telephone care as part of their curricula.

A variety of attempts to train nurses and physicians in telephone care have been described in the literature. The methods include didactic training, manuals, audiotapes, CD-ROMs, patient feedback, role playing, observation of telephone nurses, analysis of recorded calls, small-group discussions, and simulated calls. None of these methods have been shown to produce significant, persistent improvement in performance on tests in telephone care. Although lecturing is the least-effective method of teaching skills in telephone care, it is the most commonly used method. Most telephone care training has focused on improving history taking; however, no association between history-taking ability and outcome has been shown. Studies identify a lack of an organized, consistent approach to calls as a major reason for poor performance.

The most effective means of improving performance have been shown to be

1. Use of a detailed model for how to organize a clinical call
2. Use of telephone care guidelines
3. Observation of an experienced telephone care provider
4. Supervision by an experienced telephone care provider
5. Performance evaluation using performance standards

A telephone care training program should emphasize these 5 features. This chapter describes a training method that begins by defining a model call reflecting the objectives and values of your practice, then works from performance standards to orient and train telephone care providers. The chapter is divided into 3 parts: the model call, training, and special and difficult situations.

The Model Call

Defining the Model Call

The most common complaint about telephone care is that the caller must wait too long to speak to someone. The most common reason for delays is that telephone care providers spend too much time with each call. Spending too much time on calls affects not only patient satisfaction, but also the profitability of the practice. The cost of telephone care is directly proportional to call duration, and the single most significant determinant of call duration is the ability of the telephone care provider to be organized. Defining a model call for telephone care providers to use will supply the necessary structure to ensure professional, efficient, and cost-effective telephone care. For each step of the model call, define the target length of time devoted to the step and the specific actions expected of the telephone care provider. You also will want to develop explanations of the reasoning behind each step. The model call will serve as the core of your training program and allow you to integrate training, performance evaluation, quality improvement (QI), and continuing telephone care education.

Organizing the Triage and Advice Call

Each practice must decide on the components, sequence, and target times that are best suited to its practice style and philosophy. The model call is best designed in collaboration among the physicians, mid-level practitioners, telephone care providers, practice manager, and reception/scheduling staff. Table 6-1 shows an example from an urban private practice on how to organize a model call.

Table 6-1 How to Organize the Triage and Advice Call		
Component of the Call	**Target Time**	**Range**
Greeting	15 seconds	10-15 seconds
Active listening	30 seconds	30-60 seconds
Verifying demographic information	15 seconds	15-30 seconds
Assessment, chronic problems, medications, allergies	30 seconds	15-60 seconds
Triage using guidelines	2 minutes	1-3 minutes
Advice	2 minutes	1-3 minutes
Closure	30 seconds	15-120 seconds
Total	7 minutes	4-11 minutes

In this model, the telephone care provider uses the first 15 seconds to greet the caller, introduce herself, and begin to develop a relationship. The next 30 to 60 seconds are used to get a basic understanding of the problem by letting the caller describe the problem in his or her own words. Then, the provider takes more control of the call and asks the directed questions. The provider briefly verifies the demographic information of the caller and patient and asks about chronic problems, medications, and allergies. Using this initial information, supplemented by a few questions, the provider selects a telephone care guideline by identifying what appears to be the most important symptom for the patient (usually, either the most prominent or most serious symptom).

Then, the provider asks questions in the exact order provided by the symptom guideline. The telephone care provider continues to ask questions until the appropriate disposition is determined. At that point the provider proceeds to advice-giving, such as where the patient should be cared for and what the caller should do to provide appropriate care at home (including instructions on what to do if the condition of the patient changes). One of the arts of telephone care is learning to control the pace and direction of the call without asking leading questions that might distort the caller's answers. In the last phase of the call, the provider must determine if the caller has any more questions or concerns, whether the caller feels comfortable with the disposition and advice, and if the caller is able and willing to comply with the advice and direction provided.

The sequence of events in listening to the presenting complaint, obtaining demographic information, and identifying chronic diseases, medications, and allergies often has to be adjusted to the caller. Many practices prefer to verify demographic information first before allowing the caller to describe the presenting complaint. This can be a topic to discuss at a telephone care QI meeting (Chapter 14). The need for an appointment may become obvious early in some calls, allowing the telephone care provider to limit assessment and advice.

Organizing the Health Information-Only Call
Some clinical calls are for health information only (eg, medication dosages, fever control). Providing specific targeted information is appropriate for most of these calls, yet for some of them triage and advice may actually be needed. The provider should use her skills, knowledge base, and experience to recognize such situations.

The typical health information-only call takes 3 to 4 minutes, with a range of 3 to 6 minutes. The key decision is whether to simply give the information or go through the triage and advice process. Clearly, the safest approach, if there is any question about whether to do triage, is to follow the full triage and advice process. The telephone care provider should spend enough time to feel comfortable that triage and advice is not needed. The components of the health information call are detailed in Table 6-2.

Components of the Model Call

Greeting, Introduction, and Establishing a Working Relationship
The goal for providers is to identify themselves and convince the caller that they are pleasant, skilled, and willing to be of help. Callers have often struggled with the decision to call and need to hear a voice that sounds receptive and approachable. The tone of voice and demeanor

Table 6-2 How to Organize the Health Information-Only Call		
Component of the Call	**Target Time**	**Range**
Greeting, introduction, relationship	15 seconds	10-15 seconds
Active listening and presenting problem	15-30 seconds	30-60 seconds
Verifying demographic information	15 seconds	15-30 seconds
Assessment, chronic problems, medications, allergies	30 seconds	30-60 seconds
Decision whether to give information or go through triage and advice	-----------	-----------
Giving the information	2 minutes	1-3 minutes
Closure	15-30 seconds	15-60 seconds
Total	3-4 minutes	3-6 minutes

should be professional, but should also convince the caller that the telephone care provider is in a pleasant mood. Providers need to pay attention to how they sound. They should strive to not sound busy, abrupt, disinterested, unfriendly, judgmental, blaming, argumentative, too controlling, or inflexible.

It is ideal for the telephone care providers in a practice to agree on standard wording for the greeting and introduction, although some people will feel a need to modify it to fit their personalities. The greeting should identify the provider by name and role, link him or her to someone callers know and trust (eg, the primary care physician, the practice), and offer to help. For example, "Hello, this is Jane, the nurse from Denver Family Practice, calling back for Dr Smith. How can I help you today?" This open-ended offer of help shows interest and allows callers to express their concerns early. This helps callers relax. Although it is important to obtain patient demographics early in the call, it is more important to let callers explain why they are calling first. "Doctor's office" should be avoided because physicians frequently have similar numbers, and interoffice call routing systems can be confusing. It also is important to provide your answering service with a precise script for how to greet callers and notify the caller of its role.

Traditional wisdom suggests that callers should be addressed using a title and their last name. This is not the only or best option. We live in a far less formal society now and people may be addressed respectfully using their first name. Callers are far more interested in how they are treated overall than in how they are addressed. Above all, community standards and what best represents the physician's personal style should be respected.

Verifying Demographic Information

The provider should take a brief moment to verify the necessary demographic information once the caller sounds confident he or she will be treated in a pleasant, attentive, and helpful manner. It is good to let the caller describe his or her concerns before collecting the demographic data. Early in the call, however, the provider can say, "Before we talk more about the problem you are having today, let me get some information for the record of the call." This makes it easier to document the demographic information and allows the provider to obtain a telephone number and name if the call is unexpectedly disconnected.

The practice should develop a policy addressing whether to provide telephone triage and advice to nonestablished patients. If the practice wishes to provide telephone care to established patients only, the provider should verify that the caller has an established relationship with the practice.

The provider should be sure to know who called originally. When returning a call, it is very important to make certain that the provider or a representative speak with the same person who made the initial call or someone the caller would allow to represent him or her. Each family member will see the same situation differently and have different issues to discuss. The provider may still end up having to speak with the original caller and duplicate time and effort in managing the call. No matter with whom the provider speaks, it is always important to respect privacy and confidentiality of the patient.

Active Listening and Identifying the Presenting Complaint

The next step is for the provider to listen and give the caller full attention. The caller can sense when providers are distracted and trying to do too many things at once, and this distraction can lead to mistakes and decreased caller satisfaction. Providers should eliminate inappropriate and distracting background noise. Loud music or other conversations that can be overheard are not professional and may cause the provider or caller to become distracted.

Providers should always let the caller explain the purpose of the call, rather than assume they know the reason for the call. As the provider listens to the caller, the provider begins documenting the information that will be needed during the call so that it will not need to be repeated later. Initially, it is important to allow the caller to talk for 30 to 60 seconds, or even longer if the caller is providing organized, useful information that will definitely be needed. This will provide information about the caller's concerns.

The provider then identifies the most concerning symptom or problem and helps the caller be an accurate reporter. "What are you most concerned/worried about today?" The provider validates the caller's role as an observer and reporter by asking, "How concerned are you about…?"

Active listening involves clarifying what the caller is saying to be sure that the provider understands what the caller is trying to convey. The provider summarizes what is being heard and repeats it back to the caller, giving the caller the opportunity to correct or add to it. "Let me make sure I have the correct information/the full picture." "From what you are saying, it sounds as if…"

As the provider is listening, in addition to obtaining information about the patient, caller demographics, and information pertaining to determining appropriate disposition, the provider should attempt to answer the following questions:

- How anxious or concerned is the patient?
- Is this patient sophisticated enough to understand health care advice?
- Is the patient impaired in any way?
- What are the background noises, and how should it affect my actions?
- Should I ask to speak to anyone else?

If the provider recognizes that the patient is very worried, the provider should acknowledge it and express empathy. "I can tell you are very concerned, and I imagine that you didn't get much sleep last night."

Also, the provider should positively reinforce those things that the patient has done appropriately. "Well, you have taken your temperature and taken the correct dosage of ibuprofen. That is excellent." Sometimes patients call just to see if what they have done is appropriate. So telling a patient they have done a good job and to call back if they need anything else may be all that is necessary and is a good way to build a relationship.

After a brief period of active listening, the telephone care provider should take control of the flow of the communication. The provider should explain to the caller that certain questions need to be asked in a particular order to help the caller effectively. The provider should try to limit communication to only the information needed for triage.

Brief Patient Assessment, Chronic Problems, Medications, Allergies
As the provider takes charge of the call, questions to develop a systematic assessment of the patient should follow. What related symptoms need to be asked about? Enough information must be gathered during this phase of the call to ensure that the most serious and concerning symptoms will be assessed. Patients may focus on 1 or 2 symptoms and fail to mention other symptoms they feel are minor or unrelated. They may not have noticed other symptoms until you ask them to look for particular problems. This also is the time to clarify information with questions about onset, severity, degree, rate, etc. Are others in the home experiencing similar symptoms? Information about any treatment they have instituted also should be gathered. How much of what have they done? What has been the effect?

When the patient is a child, assess the child's activity level and general appearance. This often is the most useful information and will frequently have a direct relationship to the disposition. How active is the child and is the child responding to or interacting with the parent or environment? "What is he doing right now?" "What was he doing before he fell asleep?" "Tell me what Bobby has been doing for the past few hours." "Has he been playing? Watching television? Responding to you?" "Is he sitting up and drinking?" "Is he able to walk to the bathroom?" "How sick does he look to you?" Questions about infants must be age appropriate. "Will he hold a bottle?" "If you put him on the floor, will he crawl to you?" A significantly decreased activity level, a child who is not interacting with his or her environment, and/or a child who looks very sick to the caller is a child who deserves very careful triage and probably requires immediate attention.

The provider should then take another moment to ask whether the patient has any chronic illnesses, ongoing problems, regular medications, and known allergies. For practices that have the patient's medical record available at the time of the call, the steps for verifying demographics and reviewing chronic problems, medications, and allergies can be quick, but should be done just to be sure that nothing has changed.

Selecting the Appropriate Guideline

The most difficult and important step in the entire process is selecting the appropriate guideline. The provider must know what guidelines are available to select the most appropriate one for reaching a safe and reasonable disposition. For example, a patient who complains of numbness in his arm and has a cough and runny nose would not be appropriately triaged if the telephone care provider selected the runny nose or cough as the highest risk symptom to triage. Each telephone triage and advice guideline book or program has an introductory section describing how to use the guidelines. This should be read during orientation. Consult the description of how to select the best telephone care guideline described in the introduction to the guidelines that you are using.

Generally, when determining the most appropriate guideline to use, the provider

- Identifies the symptoms that the patient has recognized
- Determines which symptoms seem most prominent
- Determines which symptoms seem most serious

Then, the provider selects the guideline most likely to result in a more urgent disposition (eg, the most serious problem). This requires clinical experience. Onset, duration, and severity (frequency, intensity, amount) of the symptoms are always prime considerations. With this information in mind, the provider should select a guideline using the following parameters:

- If the patient has one predominant symptom, use that guideline.
- If there are multiple symptoms, select the most severe symptom or the one that seems most likely to be an emergency.
- For fever, use the guideline for the most serious associated symptom, unless the fever is very high (greater than 104.5°F), in which case, use the fever guideline *also.*
- *When in doubt, use more than one guideline and select the higher acuity disposition.*
- If the guideline book provides a rank order of symptoms, use that list to select the most significant symptom.

Do not accept the patient's diagnosis without verification through the use of appropriate questions. When patients feel they know the diagnosis, they are correct about one third of the time. Even when patients are health care professionals, they are correct only about one half of the time. For example, patients often misdiagnose varicella, "wheezing," and the rash of petechiae. So it is important for the telephone care provider to confirm the diagnosis using the guidelines. It also is important to respect the caller's level of training, without necessarily accepting their diagnosis. "Let me just ask a few more questions to be sure we have identified all of the problems."

Using the Guideline

After selecting the guideline, the triage process involves asking questions in the guideline to evaluate the patient's symptoms and systematically determine the appropriate disposition. The questions are usually arranged in order of acuity (severity and urgency) to reach an appropriate disposition. The initial questions are designed to identify life-threatening problems requiring mobilization of the emergency medical response system. These are followed by questions used to identify patients who need to be seen immediately. These questions are, in turn, followed by questions that identify patients who can wait until later that day to be seen and who can be seen the next day, or even later. Last are questions that identify conditions that can be managed at home without a visit. For this reason, the provider must ask questions in the exact order presented until the first positive response is obtained. Sometimes patients give information rapidly or out of order, so the provider must be flexible. The telephone care provider must *make sure all of the questions are covered* until the first positive response or until it is determined that the patient can safely be managed with home care instructions only.

To make most efficient use of the call time, the telephone care provider must direct the flow of the call and focus on the guideline questions. However, it is important to avoid asking multiple questions at the same time and asking leading questions such as "You don't have a cough, do you?" Once the disposition is determined, the appropriate, corresponding advice is given.

Deciding on the Disposition and Providing Appropriate Advice

The triage guidelines and disposition (assuming a physician in the practice has reviewed them) serve as the physician's orders. The guidelines should answer the following questions:

- Does additional evaluation need to be done at home?
- Does the patient need to see a health care provider?
- If the patient needs to be seen, how soon and in what type of setting?
- Where should the patient be cared for?
- What care advice should the provider offer?
- What are the callback criteria?

Once a disposition is reached, it should be discussed with the caller. The provider should make certain that the caller understands the basic reason for the disposition. If a "911" disposition is reached, the provider must quickly tell the caller what to do. The provider should determine if the caller agrees with the level of concern. Does the provider need to say more to convince the caller or say less and get off the phone so that emergency medical services (EMS) can be activated? Who will call EMS? What should be done in the meantime? If the provider decides on a lesser disposition but the patient needs to be seen, the provider should explain when that should happen and where. What should be done in the meantime? If the patient is likely to respond to home care, the provider should offer appropriate suggestions for care, giving the patient a chance to write down the suggestions and ask questions.

In other situations, the provider should always let the caller know what to expect. Is someone going to call him or her back? When? Today? Around what time? Will a prescription be called in? When? The provider should never assume the caller knows the policies or timetables.

Every caller should be made aware if prescriptions are routinely called in at a specific time or if callbacks are made at certain times of the day. Busy professionals need an opportunity to plan for a callback. Parents have to leave home at times in spite of the fact they have a sick child at home. This should not be treated as unreasonable behavior. Letting the caller know what to expect can cut down on repeat phone calls, upset caregivers, and missed communications. Much of this may be information that can be provided to new clients in the form of printed or Web site information about your office and practice.

Giving Callback Instructions and Leaving Access Open

A very important aspect of telephone care is the caller's need to know how to recognize worsening of the patient's condition. Callback instructions are very important clinically and medicolegally. If there are more than 2 conditions to watch for, ask the caller to write them down. The following are examples of ways to leave access open with the caller and help safeguard the health of patients: "If these symptoms develop, please call me back." "If you become more concerned, please call me." "If you feel worse in any way, please call." "Call back if you don't see improvement within…(specify a time period)." "Feel free to call back."

Bringing Closure to the Call

The end of the call is devoted to identifying and handling any problems, concerns, or barriers to the care recommended. The telephone care provider assesses the caller's willingness and ability to carry out the care recommendations.

- Does the patient understand the disposition and advice? Ask the patient to repeat his or her understanding, if you have any concerns.
- Does the patient know what to do, what to look for, and when to call back?
- Is the caller comfortable with the advice?
- Is the caller willing to follow the advice?
- Suggest that the caller write down critical instructions (such as medication dosages or parameters for callback).
- Be certain that the patient is able to carry out the plan (no logistic barriers such as transportation issues, other responsibilities, disabilities, or money).

Ask the caller to describe how he or she is feeling about the disposition and advice. Acknowledge the patient's anxiety and accommodate his or her needs for more information or reassurance. If the caller cannot be reassured, arrange for him or her to speak to a physician or to be seen. If the problem seems minor and the patient is uncomfortable, arrange for a follow-up call in 1 to 2 hours. Anxious patients who are not accommodated become a much higher liability risk.

Often callers have more than one concern, and sometimes there is reluctance to mention the second concern ("hidden agendas" or "overlooked concerns"). "Is there anything we haven't covered?" "Is there anything more you want to tell me?" "Is there anything else I should know?" "Is there anything else you wanted to ask me?"

If pressed for time, at least ask the following questions at the end of each call: "Do you feel as though you understand what I am recommending?" "Do you have any questions?" "Are you feeling comfortable with the advice you have received?" "Do you think you will have any problems following this advice?"

Follow-up Calls

Some guidelines recommend follow-up calls. Most do not. Patients are very grateful for the follow-up. It conveys interest and concern. Decide whether you want to do follow-up calls on a routine basis. Most practices will decide not to. If the telephone care provider feels uncomfortable with a particular situation, then a callback is warranted. Consider developing policies about the more serious situations in which a follow-up call may be helpful. You will do fewer follow-up calls as you gain experience.

Additional Calls

Additional calls associated with the case may take extra time (eg, calls to arrange for the patient to be seen by another office or emergency department [ED], calls to a pharmacy). The target time for these extra calls should be 2 to 3 minutes.

Documentation

To keep call duration short, documentation is done during the call. Chapter 4 describes the rationale for documenting all clinical calls and what information to collect and where it should be kept. During training it is important to remind new telephone care providers of the old adage, "If it is not recorded, it did not happen." Be brief. Use checklists. Use standard abbreviations. Proper documentation includes

- Demographic information: caller name, relationship and phone number, patient name and date of birth, age, date and time
- Clinical information: reason for call, presenting complaint, main symptoms (1-2 sentences or phrases)
- Guideline(s) used and pertinent positives on the questions in the guideline(s)
- Disposition recommended by the guideline
- Advice given (it is acceptable to write "per guideline"), dosages, and callback instructions (can write "per guideline")
- Caller understanding and acceptance of advice
- Signature

Training

As described previously, the most effective means of training and improving performance in telephone care have been shown to be

- Use of a detailed model explaining how to organize a clinical call
- Use of telephone care guidelines
- Observation of an experienced telephone care provider during training
- Supervision by an experienced telephone care provider
- Performance evaluation using performance standards

This section describes the ideal training process. Many factors may limit the ability of practices to meet this ideal, so they will have to adapt the process to their particular situation.

Building Commitment to the Process

Changing to a more standardized approach to telephone care can be difficult for experienced telephone care staff. It may appear to them that their experience is being undervalued or distrusted. Also, they may feel that the training period will add hours to their work and the new system will lengthen calls and force them to change. It helps to acknowledge their feelings and validate your trust in them as you discuss the goals and benefits of using a standardized approach to telephone care. This includes the use of well-researched and tested guidelines. By standardizing care, they will reduce medicolegal risk, make documentation easier, and help the office comply with upcoming standards (they will be ahead of the game). It will also make training new staff much easier.

The Training Process

Orientation and education of telephone care providers requires an experienced telephone care provider. A practice that is starting a new telephone care system may need to send its first telephone care provider to an experienced practice or medical call center for training or bring an experienced trainer to its site.

Training will focus on teaching the telephone care provider how to successfully perform each of the requirements of the model call. The following steps are recommended for the training process:

- Orientation by the trainer
- Study of specific written materials (especially this chapter)
- Trainee observation of an experienced provider for 8 hours
- Trainee closely supervised by experienced provider for several shifts
- Ongoing supervision of trainee with periodic direct observation (using performance standards) until performance goals are met (experienced provider close at hand for 1-3 months)
- Physician backup at all times (description of how to appropriately use physician backup)
- Ongoing participation in the QI process

The trainer provides an orientation that includes a review of the model call (including specific actions and target times for each step); review of the information in chapters 2 through 4, 6, 11, and 14 (with emphasis on this chapter); review of policies, procedures, and standards of performance; provision of important management tips; teaching of the use of resource materials; and review of the overall training process. The trainer shows examples of adapting the model call to common call scenarios. After the orientation, the trainer allows the trainee to observe her on the job for at least 8 hours. Then, the trainer observes the trainee for 8 to 16 hours, offering suggestions as necessary. Each telephone care provider learns at a different rate, so the duration of these first steps should depend on the progress made by the trainee. It is important to evaluate the trainee's progress during this part of the process using materials from Chapter 7. Praise the new trainee for the things that she is learning quickly and spend additional time in areas she finds more challenging.

Carefully select and prepare the materials that your trainee will be expected to read and use. The clearer and more useful these materials are the more quickly your trainee will progress.

The following should be considered as required reading for trainees:

- Chapters 2 through 4, 6, 11, and 14 in this manual. If they are going to provide after-hours telephone care, they should also read chapters 20 and 22.

- The 20 most frequently used telephone care guidelines.
- The practice's telephone care policies and procedures.
- The practice's telephone performance standards.

Other Resources

There are several books available commercially that include telephone care guidelines and orientation material for telephone care providers that can be used for training.

- *Telephone Medicine: Triage and Training for Primary Care,* 2nd Edition
  (by Harvey Katz, published by F. A. Davis Co, 2001)
- *Telephone Triage: Theory, Practice, and Protocol Development* (by Sheila Q. Wheeler
  and Judith H. Windt, published by Delmar Publishers, 1993)
- *Pediatric Telephone Protocols: Office Version,* 9th Edition (by Barton Schmitt, available
  from the American Academy of Pediatrics, 2002)
- *Pediatric Telephone Medicine: Principles, Triage, and Advice,* 2nd Edition
  (by Jeffrey L. Brown, published by Lippincott Williams and Wilkins, 1994)
- *Telephone Triage Protocols for Infants and Children: Birth to 6 Years*
  (by Sheila Q. Wheeler, published by Aspen Publishers, 1997)

Standards of Performance and Evaluation

Begin the evaluation and review process early. It is easier to devote ample time to the initial steps in the training process (especially a prolonged period of close observation) than to have to work on undoing bad habits developed because of receiving too little training. The trainer can use the evaluation materials described in Chapter 7 to evaluate and provide feedback while observing the trainee.

The standards of performance are a list of criteria by which the telephone provider will be evaluated at regular intervals to determine how well she is meeting the needs of the patients, callers, and practice. (See Chapter 7.) They include the expectations and targets for each element of the model call. These criteria are part of the job description.

The performance standards should be reviewed during training and used to provide feedback during the period of close observation by the trainer. The new telephone care provider should be observed on a regular basis by the trainer (even after the first or second shift) until the time when the new provider is able to meet all of the performance standards. At any time, whether during training or later, if the provider does not meet these standards, it should trigger an automatic return to the training process. The provider should review appropriate materials, observe an accomplished provider who is meeting this standard, be observed by the telephone care manager who should provide suggestions, and be evaluated again within a month.

The trainer also should review a sample of the trainee's log sheets at the end of 1, 3, and 6 months to provide feedback. After that, ongoing review for all telephone care providers should occur on a regular basis. (See Chapter 7.) A very important element in the learning process is receiving feedback based on the outcome of the patient. It is very helpful to see the patient or hear about how the patient actually looked on arrival, particularly for telephone care providers who are new to telephone triage. (See Chapter 14.) All telephone care providers also should participate in periodic educational sessions to discuss interesting or difficult calls and should participate in quality assurance sessions. (See Chapter 14.)

The Most Important Skills

Many important skills are involved in providing excellent telephone care. The skill that most affects the efficiency of telephone care is the effective organization of the call. Appropriate guideline selection and use influences quality of care. Manner, etiquette, and listening skills most influence caller satisfaction. Closure skills highly influence outcome and medicolegal risk. The length of the call has a direct influence on the cost of care. Critical thinking skills are important throughout the call process. The critical decision points for the telephone care provider include

- Selecting the appropriate telephone care guideline
- Recognizing and recommending the correct disposition
- Ensuring that the caller feels comfortable with the disposition and advice

These skills are the most important in determining the safe, effective outcome for the patient, and they are the most difficult elements to teach and practice. For this reason these topics deserve the greatest attention during the initial orientation and the shifts in which the trainee observes another telephone care provider or is closely supervised. These skills require emphasis and repetition during training.

Using the Guidelines

To get a feel for using the guidelines, the trainee should select one (eg, fever) and study it, noting how the first questions identify the most serious symptoms. She can imagine what would happen if she skipped some of the initial questions. She should study the top 20 guidelines to get a feel for the questions. Telephone care providers should be taught to adhere to guideline-driven dispositions unless their clinical judgment causes them to question the disposition.

There may be times when the telephone care provider does not feel comfortable with the disposition recommended by the telephone care guideline. The telephone care provider should be taught not to suggest a disposition to a lower level of health care, unless she confers with a physician. If the telephone care provider feels that the disposition should be upgraded to a higher level of care (sooner or more urgent), she also may want advice from a physician. *There should be a low threshold for consulting the backup physician.*

If the telephone care provider feels that communication is not effective (for any reason, including language difference, cultural differences, caller's ability to comprehend, or unhelpful attitudes), the patient should be seen. Factors that may cause a telephone care provider to reconsider the disposition include

- Reliability of the caller as observer
- Effectiveness of the caller as communicator or reporter
- The caller's ability to follow through with care advice
- The caller's comfort with care plan
- Potential logistical barriers to care (eg, availability of a car, distance from care)
- Symptoms seem vague
- Chronic illness

Overriding the Guideline Disposition

Experienced registered nurses who are using good telephone care guidelines override the disposition in 1 out of 20 to 25 calls. The override may be in the direction of more or less intervention. When a telephone care nurse overrides guidelines it is to suggest more intervention (seeing the patient sooner) 75% to 80% of the time. The provider may have a sense that the patient is more ill than the guideline was able to determine. In this instance the provider is encouraged to follow her intuition. Override rates should be tracked to be sure that they do not exceed 5%. When a provider feels inclined to override the guideline toward less intervention (a less common event), the provider should check with the physician. When in doubt, have the patient seen.

Patients express their discomfort with the disposition or advice around 5% of the time. When patients request a higher level of intervention, it is most sensible to accommodate their request, from a caller satisfaction and medicolegal standpoint. When they request a lower level of intervention than recommended by the guidelines, it is wise to have the caller speak to a physician.

Use Your Physician Backup

Highly experienced telephone care providers consult physicians on perhaps 5% to 10% of office hours telephone care calls. Consult a physician

- When the guideline recommends it
- If you, for any reason, cannot completely evaluate the problem over the phone
- If you feel uncomfortable with the caller or disposition
- If the caller demands it
- If you are unsure which guideline to use

Giving Advice

Telephone care guidelines recommend specific advice for the caller depending on the disposition. The telephone care provider should provide the advice recommended in the guideline, unless it has been adapted during the review process by the practice medical director. In giving advice, always use language that the caller can understand. Medical terminology is often misunderstood or not understood at all by callers. This can lead to distraction or confusion. Calling a sore throat "pharyngitis" may be appropriate for a patient's chart, but not for a conversation with most patients. While they are trying to figure out what you just said they are missing the next part of your conversation. If there are more than 2 things to remember, ask the caller to write down the advice. Make sure that the advice is clear and easy to follow. Patients should repeat medication forms and dosages to prevent errors. If there is any question about the caller's understanding of the advice, ask the caller to repeat the advice. Ask the caller if he or she understands the advice. Ask if there will be any problems in implementing the recommendations.

Telephone care providers should not refer to family remedies or themselves. For example, do not say, "I have tried _____ and it seems to work."

Taking care of a person who is sick can be hard work, and callers appreciate knowing that you recognize and applaud their efforts. Always find something about which you can compliment and encourage the caller. It is never appropriate to make patients or the person who calls on their behalf feel guilty. If you would like to see different behavior next time the patient is sick, make forward-looking statements such as "in the future" or "if this happens again you can…." Keep the language and tone of the call positive.

Medication Management

Every practice should have a policy on the telephone care provider's management of medications, both prescription and nonprescription drugs (Chapter 9). The policies should be reviewed by a physician in the practice. When are medications recommended? What medications can be recommended over the phone? What dosage tables will be used? What prescriptions are refilled? All of these policies must comply with all appropriate state and federal regulations.

For example, there should be a specific policy about the recommendation of rescue medications in the telephone management of asthma that ensures patients are seen for more severe symptoms, worsening symptoms, unresponsive symptoms, or frequent acute episodes. Medication management may not be adequately addressed in the telephone care guidelines, so this is another reason a physician should review all guidelines.

Doses of medication for children often are given on a milligram per kilogram or pound basis. Although it is helpful to have dosage charts available for use by the telephone care providers, there will be times when calculations of dosages will have to be made. It is crucial that this skill be practiced during the initial training session for the common over-the-counter (OTC) medications acetaminophen, ibuprofen, pseudoephedrine, dextromethorphan, and diphenhydramine. The provider also should become familiar with the dosage formats.

Example: Weight 17 lb. The dose for acetaminophen infant drops (80 mg/0.8 mL) is 7 mg/lb/dose, so 7 x 17 = 119 mg. To convert the volume of the liquid:

$$119 \text{ mg} \times \frac{0.8 \text{ mL}}{80 \text{ mg}} = 1.19 \text{ mL}$$

which is close to 1.2 mL or $1\frac{1}{2}$ infant dropperfuls every 4 hours as needed.

It is very helpful to have dosage tables that show the appropriate dose of common OTC medications by the weight of the child. However, the telephone care provider needs to be able to calculate doses accurately. Documentation of medication management should be complete and timely.

Goals for Call Duration

Although the telephone care provider's first priority is to provide competent care for the patient, the next responsibility is to do so in a time-efficient manner. The following are ways to improve the time efficiency of the call:

- Have a realistic call time target. (See Table 6-1.)
- Know the guidelines.
- If the caller wants an appointment, do not do triage. Simply schedule an appointment.
- Direct the conversation.
- When appropriate, give information by fax, e-mail, mail, or printed or Web-based information.
- Use brief documentation (eg, advice "per guideline").
- Avoid counseling or handling complex problems. If you cannot give the advice in 5 minutes, schedule an appointment for the patient.

The new telephone care provider is seldom able to meet all of the target times for the elements of the model call during the early weeks and months; however, by 3 to 6 months, she should be able to. A 3- and 6-month evaluation can be helpful in identifying ways to better organize calls.

Ongoing Training

One of the most common reasons nurses leave the private practice setting is lack of opportunity to learn new things. Promote the attitude that the practice is interested in learning and improving, as opposed to criticizing and finding fault. Therefore, everyone learns every day in the practice, and everyone assists each other in learning by sharing interesting calls or insights. Training continues for everyone in the QI process in addition to regular telephone care meetings. (See Chapter 14.)

If a telephone care provider's evaluation is not up to standard, then a plan for retraining should be developed that involves reviewing written material in the area needing improvement, practicing the needed skills while being observed, and being reevaluated after a period of practice and observation.

Other Key Points to Remember

Do not assume the patient is not very sick. Most acute illnesses in adults and children are not very serious, so there is a tendency among providers to assume that the situation is not serious. However, the provider's role is to carefully determine in each instance whether a situation is serious. Avoid stereotyping callers. Be rigorous about asking standard questions for each call. Use physician backup.

Consult a physician if

- The guideline recommends it.
- You are unable to completely evaluate the problem over the phone.
- You feel uncomfortable with the caller or disposition.
- The caller demands it.
- You are unsure of the guideline to use.
- The patient has a complex chronic disease.

Know the regulations about nursing practice in your state. In most states, by law, nurses, medical assistants, and health assistants do not make diagnoses; they make nursing assessments and then recommend dispositions based on that assessment. Generally, they are allowed to prescribe only certain medications, and only by protocol. All telephone care providers need to be familiar with the regulations in their state and stay within them. This usually means developing office protocols for calling in medication prescriptions and for when to consult a physician.

Patients often assume that the telephone care provider can develop a complete and accurate diagnosis of their problem over the phone. In most states, it is important to carefully state what you are doing within the state regulations. The telephone care provider needs to be clear that she has done a nursing assessment and based on that limited information is recommending a disposition. The care provider needs to emphasize that the assessment and disposition is based on the symptoms at the time of the call and may change as the illness changes.

"From what you have told me, it sounds as though you do not need to see a physician at this time. Let me make some suggestions for caring for yourself. If things change...."

Maintain confidentiality. Callers should always be assured that their disclosures will be treated professionally. Information should be shared only as needed (the billing staff does not need to know that a parent is experiencing postpartum depression). Conversely, in professional management of information, you should never agree to withhold information from other professional staff in your office who also provide care to your patient. A nonphysician provider must always be free to share significant information with the physician.

Avoid communication equipment problems. Caller ID blocks on the caller's home phone when the provider is returning a call can be a problem. The solution is to ask the answering service to remind patients to unblock their phones. A reminder also can be put in the practice telephone policy and on voice messages in the automated telephone attendant for callers to unblock their phones when they are waiting for a return call from the practice.

Remain candid. Always be truthful with the caller. If the doctor is running late, say so. If the provider is not in yet, mention it. If you do not know the answer to a question, be honest with the caller. Do you need time to do some checking or research? Tell the caller. If someone in the office fails to act appropriately, it is reasonable to apologize. No one expects perfection, but people do expect fairness, honesty, respect, and consideration.

Training Reception/Scheduling Staff

It is current conventional wisdom that reception/scheduling staff should not be expected to do telephone triage and advice. However, when patients call in for an appointment, it is inevitable that the receptionist/scheduler and caller will have to decide whether to arrange an urgent appointment or whether the problem can wait until a later appointment is available. In some instances, neither the patient nor the receptionist will have enough knowledge to make that decision. Each practice must struggle with the dilemma of how to deal with this situation.

The most common telephone care malpractice cases involve a patient calling an office in the morning for an acute illness appointment and neither the patient nor the receptionist recognizing the urgency of the problem so the patient is given a late-day or next-day appointment. The patient's illness progresses while waiting to be seen resulting in a serious condition with an avoidable poor outcome. Each practice should discuss this problem as a group and decide how to prevent such a situation. One strategy is to provide the reception/scheduling staff with a list of conditions that should be handled quickly by the telephone care provider or physician (the red-flag list). This list should include conditions shown in Table 6-3.

The most conservative approach is to have all other calls for an acute problem that cannot be worked into the office schedule within 4 hours be passed along to the telephone care provider. It is important for the reception/scheduling staff to feel comfortable in consulting the nurse or physician if there is any question.

The solution to this problem will vary depending on the size of the practice, training and experience of various staff members, and level of involvement of physicians and mid-level practitioners in telephone care. Whatever the practice decides about this dilemma should be expressed in a policy and become part of the training of all staff.

Table 6-3
Emergent Conditions

- Difficulty breathing (choking, stopped breathing, weak breathing, stridor, blue)

- Possible anaphylaxis (difficulty breathing or swallowing following medicine, bee stings, eating)

- Neurologic symptoms (seizure, loss of consciousness, hard to awaken, confusion)

- Poisoning, ingestion, or drug overdose

- Trauma to the neck or eye

- Uncontrollable bleeding

- Suicide threats or attempts and rape/abuse calls

- Fever in an infant younger than 3 months

- Fever greater than 104.5°F

- Inconsolable crying

- Chest pain

- Severe pain

- Near drowning

- Penetrating wounds

- Very anxious caller

- Head trauma with behavior change or recurrent vomiting

- Purple or blood-colored rash

The reception/scheduling staff should

- Be required to read the telephone policy book.
- Understand the components of the model call for telephone care and the triage and advice process so they can assist the telephone care provider in obtaining needed information.
- Memorize the red-flag list.
- Have a low threshold to turn a call over to the telephone care provider.
- Understand the caller satisfaction standards.

Difficult Calls and Special Situations

Difficult Callers

There will always be difficult calls and callers. It is important that providers learn to handle these calls without escalating the difficulty of the call. One of the most helpful approaches is to accept that these types of calls are part of dealing with the public, and that we all receive them from time to time. Difficult callers can include angry, overly worried, difficult to understand, or impaired callers. Each of these situations requires specific techniques to increase the likelihood of a satisfactory outcome. It is helpful to develop practice policies that describe how your practice staff will respond to these types of callers. (See Chapter 9.)

The Angry or Frustrated Caller

This is often the most feared call. The instinctive responses are to become either defensive and angry or to feel overpowered because these callers raise their voices, threaten, or make demands. Both of these responses reduce the likelihood of a good outcome for the call. A better beginning is to recognize that we all get angry at times. We all occasionally encounter situations that frustrate us beyond our ability to cope with them in our usual manner. Most angry callers are frustrated callers. They have tried to work through our "system," and they have become frustrated. In some situations people have made repeated attempts to take care of the problem, and resolution is no closer. In other instances, patients are tired or frightened because of their illness. At other times, their anger or frustration has little to do with us. We were simply the proverbial "last straw."

Begin by acknowledging the callers' feelings or state of mind. Statements such as "I can tell you are upset" immediately followed by a sincere offer to help will usually diffuse the callers' anger or frustration. They are finally getting what they had hoped for—HELP! Avoid telling callers that you can tell they are angry. Many people recognize it is acceptable to be frustrated or upset but are not comfortable with being told they are angry. Allow the callers to tell you why they are frustrated. Listen thoughtfully, and then try to move the callers forward with what can be done now. "Mr Johnson, I am sorry things didn't work as you had wanted before, but the important thing now is to get the prescription called in. Give me 5 minutes and I will call you back to confirm that has been done." Who can best help them? How quickly will someone help them? ("Mrs Taylor, Susan handles laboratory results. She is in a room with a patient right now. Tell me the number where we can call you in the next 20 minutes and I assure you that you will receive a call.") Be specific, promise action, and then deliver what you have promised. Most callers respond positively if they understand that someone is taking the situation seriously and that there is progress toward getting needs met. Families expect competent, considerate care, which includes honesty and respect. If the caller is due an apology, then apologize. It helps and is the right thing to do.

Abusive Callers

There are callers who are angry or upset that cross a line and become abusive. Those callers are dealt with differently. Abusive callers include those whose language is clearly unacceptable, those attacking the character of the provider or someone else in the organization, and those threatening inappropriate action. No one should tolerate that behavior. Record or document the exact content of the call. Warn the caller that his or her behavior is inappropriate and you cannot help him or her if the particular behavior continues. If the behavior continues and you are not the primary care physician, tell the caller you are going to hang up and have the physician return the call. It is never appropriate to hang up on a caller unless you warn him or her you are going to terminate the call and give a reason. ("Mr Johnson, we are obviously not going to agree on this. We do not seem to be making any progress. I think we need to think about this and talk again later. I am going to hang up now, but I will call you tomorrow.") Ask the caller how he or she can be reached. Notify the physician as soon as possible. If you are the physician, let the caller know that the behavior is unacceptable and needs to change if the relationship is to be maintained. Do not fail to care for the patient appropriately. If the behavior does not change, consider following your state law concerning asking the family to find another provider. If a caller ever threatens to harm you or anyone else, notify the proper authority immediately—no exceptions. The only exception to the policy of not terminating a call without warning, reason, and a plan is the obscene caller. You should hang up on these callers immediately.

The Very Worried Caller
All practitioners receive calls from very worried callers. Those caring for children in their practices can expect many of them. Adults who normally are calm and confident may become anxious and unsure when ill or injured. Adults who may be very rational and comfortable managing their own illness may not be able to be as comfortable and rational about illness in another family member. Many of these callers are the parents of young children or first-time parents. There are 4 main factors that can contribute to the caller's concerns.

Lack of Experience or Knowledge
First-time parents trying to manage a new symptom their child is experiencing, whether it is a common or uncommon problem, are likely to call. Some parents have had very little experience with parenting or watching others parent and want your help. For these parents, every new symptom will be a challenge. They view you as their partner in caring for their child, and they want and need your assistance. Acknowledge and accept that they have little experience. Let them know that your practice is available to help them gain experience and confidence.

Information Overload
We may live in the information age, but most of us recognize that not all information is created equal. Not all information is reliable. Patients are bombarded with "medical" information and advice from relatives, neighbors, friends, teachers, television, radio, etc, whether they seek it or not. For those who seek additional information, there are books, videos, classes, pamphlets, and the Internet. Statistics suggest that approximately 80% of Internet users have sought medical information at some time. All of this would imply that patients are better educated when, in reality, patients may actually be more confused and less confident because they encounter conflicting and incomplete information and data. You may need to help them discern which information is reliable. Many of us fail to realize that information is not the complete health care tool. It is the application of that knowledge that patients sometimes find difficult. We have all had that student experience of knowing textbook information and parameters, passing the test, but lacking confidence in the early application of that knowledge

in a practical setting. Patients often seek confirmation that they are doing the right thing and that things are moving in the right direction.

Inability to Understand Complex Information

Some callers are less able than others to handle somewhat complex information. These callers may or may not recognize their limitations but have difficulty managing out-of-the-ordinary situations, including their illnesses. Accurately assessing this is important but may be difficult. Always consider seeing the patient if you cannot get clear, concise, complete information. Directions for these patients need to be simple, direct, and short-term. Instructions should not contain too many "ifs." Ask callers to paraphrase your instructions to check their understanding. ("Tell me how much medicine you will give your child.") Avoid asking closed-ended questions about their understanding. ("Do you understand these instructions?") Check on this patient frequently. Beginning-of-the-day and end-of-the-day calls to these patients may avoid after-hours calls or unnecessary ED visits.

Guilt

Sometimes a caller seems overly worried because he or she feels guilty. Patients may feel guilty about not following medical advice given previously. Other callers may be driven by guilt from other sources. A parent or caregiver who has not sought care in a timely manner, who works outside the home, or who has a chronically ill child or has experienced the loss of a child may seem overly concerned about seemingly minor symptoms. This is another instance in which it is important to express understanding and provide advice in a way that does not increase the caregiver's guilt. Anything that helps to build a caregiver's confidence may lead to better care for your patient.

The Financially Disadvantaged Caller

Sometimes calls or callers become difficult because of financial obstacles faced in providing care. Patients may agree with our recommendations but may feel that they face insurmountable financial obstacles in providing the recommended care. It is difficult to predict which callers might disclose that they cannot afford a prescription medication, an ED visit, or another proposed modality of care. We have heard these types of concerns from the uninsured caller, the suddenly unemployed caller, the insured caller with a very high deductible, the caller who is on vacation and out of network, and the caller who is not certain that his or her insurance will cover the service. While it is not our responsibility to solve people's financial problems, there are times when treatment approaches can be adjusted without endangering a patient. Is it possible to try home care for 2 more hours to see if we can get things "turned around" before a patient has to go to the ED? Can a patient come to the office now even though you usually do not see patients after 4:00 pm? Does the child with a temperature of 102°F really have to have acetaminophen? It can be difficult for all involved when a caller discloses his or her in-ability to afford services, but we actually should be grateful that the caller has been honest with us, and tell the caller. It is important to know when our advice or recommendations will not be followed.

When patients face an expense for which they are not prepared, and you feel there are no other treatment options, it is important that patients understand that you have considered their financial situation and that your recommendation is unchanged. A caring discussion with callers about doing the right thing now for the patient and worrying about the finances later will usually turn the situation around. Never threaten patients, but make certain they understand why you are concerned and include enough information about possible adverse outcomes to make sure they understand the situation is a potentially serious one.

The Caller Who Speaks a Foreign Language

As our culture becomes increasingly diverse, we encounter callers for whom English is not their first language. These callers' English skills will range from excellent to very poor. Those callers with very poor skills will present the greatest challenge, but it is important to remember that there is an increased risk of miscommunication with any of these callers. There are several things that we can do to decrease that risk.

Respect the Effort the Caller Is Making

Learning a new culture and language is a formidable task. Some callers progress quickly, others do not. Do your best to assist them. Does anyone in the office speak his or her language? It may be possible that another staff member could speak to the caller even though it may not be his or her usual role.

Encourage the Caller to Try

Many callers doubt their ability to communicate adequately, but their skills are better than they think. Ask them to try to speak with you. Tell them that you will help them. Many times you will actually be able to manage the call despite the language barriers. Speak slowly, ask one simple question at a time, and listen patiently. Encourage the caller as you move through the call. Remember that most callers understand more English than they can speak, so you may need to help fill in some of the details and ask for confirmation. Ask questions more than one way to be assured you are getting a correct picture of your patient's problem. Having tried this, if you cannot communicate with this caller, ask if someone else in the home speaks English. Be sure to establish a policy on this issue (Chapter 9).

Use a Translator

Have a well-thought-out plan for those callers with whom you are unable to communicate. If you are in an office, the hospital may have staff who can help you. There may be a local community group that provides that service. If possible, it is best to use a translator who has special skills in medical translation. There are national translation services for speakers of any language available through major telephone service providers. Learn to access these services before you need them.

Turn Off the Timer

Many of us work with formal or informal productivity expectations or we have an "internal" timer that causes us to become impatient with lengthy calls. This is another one of those calls in which the timer needs to be turned off. This is a high-risk call and must be handled as such.

Have the Patient Seen

Communicating with a caller who speaks English as a second language is a high-risk situation. If you are uncertain that your information or assessment is reliable, it is safest to see the patient.

Cultural Practices

Unless all of your services are provided to a single ethnic or cultural group, it is important to recognize the various cultural practices and approaches to health care you may encounter as you deal with members of various cultural groups in your area. When a person seeks medical care, where he or she goes and who makes the decisions are in part determined by cultural heritage. People's views reflect their own experiences and their understanding about why disease occurs and how it is best managed. These perspectives affect what we think of as disease, what we eat and drink during an illness, how we dress when we are sick, and even whether we will take a medicine or submit to a laboratory test.

Cultural practices also influence when patients call their health care providers and how they speak on the phone. For some cultures, the caller will generally be male. That male caller may not be the primary caregiver, so his information will be somewhat limited. We need to be patient while he gathers information from the caregiver. In other instances, your caller may be a very focused and careful listener who speaks slowly and expects that his or her words will be given very serious consideration. Callers from some cultures are typically loud and demanding. This does not indicate anger, but rather that they think the situation is very important. Some callers will say "yes" to anything you suggest to appear respectful, not to indicate agreement.

The variety of cultural situations we encounter grows as our population becomes more diverse. We must familiarize ourselves with the practices of those we are most likely to encounter. There is no person better able to tell us about those practices than a health care provider with a similar cultural background. Consider inviting a cultural speaker to your setting to discuss telephone management and other health care issues. The information can be very helpful and you are sending an important message to your staff about the importance of considering cultural and ethnic issues when communicating with your families.

The Caller Who Is Speech Impaired

Some callers may be difficult to understand because of a speech impediment or because they use assistive devices to amplify or synthesize speech. Give the caller your full attention. If you have difficulty understanding a caller, tell him or her you are having some problems understanding what he or she is telling you. State, "What you are telling me is important, and I want to make certain I get the correct information. I am having some difficulty understanding you, so I may have to ask you to repeat some of the information." These callers know they can be difficult to understand and are generally willing to work with you if you let them know that you sincerely want to assist them. Repeat what you understand them to be saying. "Mrs Carlson, I understand you're saying that Kathy has a temperature of 102°F, an earache, and a cough. Is that correct?" Give the caller a simple opportunity to confirm the information before you proceed. If you continue to have difficulty understanding the caller and cannot establish reliable communication, consider having someone else talk with the caller. Explain to the caller that you are still having difficulty, and that the information is very important, so you are asking another member of your staff to talk with him or her. Tell your other provider what you do understand and have confirmed with the caller so that information will not have to be repeated. If no one is able to understand the caller, offer an appointment or ask him or her to come to the office and talk with you if no one else is able to speak for him or her. Face-to-face conversations sometimes solve the communication challenge.

The Caller Who Is Hearing Impaired

Callers who are hearing impaired may contact you using a service of their phone company that allows them to type their communication. A special operator who serves as an intermediary between you and the caller will contact you. The operator's role will be to read you the caller's communication and type your response so the caller can read it. Speak as if you were talking directly to the caller. Keep your questions and directions simple so that communication remains clear and understandable. Take a moment for the basics. Introduce yourself and be certain that you know with whom you are "speaking." Before the call ends, be certain both of you agree on an action plan. When should the caller call you back? Remember that you can call this patient also. Record in the patient's chart how to contact the family using the appropriate telephone service. Develop a practice policy for this situation (Chapter 9).

The Caller Who Is Chemically Impaired

Alcohol and/or drug use, whether illegal, prescription, or OTC, may all cause mental impairment. People whose judgment or communication is impaired by the use of these substances may call you. Consider chemical impairment if your caller has slurred speech, cannot answer simple questions in a consistent manner, cannot focus on the process, seems emotionally inappropriate, or demonstrates behavior inconsistent with previous interactions. Some callers may tell you they have been drinking or have taken medication that is causing them to have difficulty talking with you but that they are concerned enough about their illness that they felt they needed to call anyway. Others may not recognize they are impaired.

When the caller is not the patient, it is important to establish early in the call that the patient is safe and likely to remain safe. Is another adult who is not impaired present? Is an older teenager there? Can you talk with that person? Can you assess the patient over the phone? Can the caller bring the patient to the phone? If the patient is capable, can he or she talk with you? It is critically important to care for your patient in the safest way possible. Can someone be notified to go to the home to help with the patient's care—a relative or friend? Never tell a caller whom you suspect to be chemically impaired to drive anywhere. It also is not advisable to ask the caller to give any nonessential medications. There is too high a risk that the medication, dosage, or frequency might be misunderstood.

Chapter 7

Standards of Performance and Performance Evaluation

The objective of performance evaluation is usually thought to be the determination of salary increases, bonuses, or promotions. While this is necessary, another more important objective of performance evaluation is to recognize the employee's skills that need improvement to plan additional training. Evaluating performance also helps to improve quality of care, reduce medicolegal risk, and ensure caller satisfaction. Performance evaluation begins during training and continues at certain intervals thereafter.

Setting the Tone

One of the most difficult responsibilities in family practice is telephone triage and advice. It carries a high level of malpractice risk and is stressful. The physician is delegating this high level of responsibility and stress to the telephone care provider. There is often pressure to handle the triage and advice calls quickly, and usually feedback comes only when there is a problem. The practice should avoid the tendency to create a high-pressure position in which there is mostly negative feedback. One way to avoid this is to define a model clinical call and have training focus on learning the skills needed to implement the model call. The evaluation process can then focus on evaluating how well the telephone care provider implements the components of the model call. The telephone care provider will receive praise and appreciation for the many successful calls handled (consistent with the model call) and for success in mastering each component of the model call. Unsuccessful calls or difficulty mastering a component of the model call becomes the focus for ongoing training and education. The focus is on what needs to be learned. Another way to set a positive tone for performance evaluation is to make it clear in the salary and organizational structure that telephone care is a highly valued role in the practice.

Standards of Performance

The standards of performance are a list of criteria by which the telephone care provider will be evaluated at regular intervals to determine how well she is meeting the needs of the patients, callers, and practice. They are reviewed in detail during training and are part of the job description. While the practice will have other performance standards for providers that relate to the other aspects of their role in the practice, following are the types of standards that may be considered for their role in providing telephone triage and advice.

The new telephone care provider will complete all of the steps in the training process. The following steps should be part of her performance standards:

1. Read chapters 2, 3, 4, 6, 11, and 14 in this manual; the top 20 telephone care guidelines; the practice's telephone care policies and procedures; and the practice's telephone care performance standards.
2. Receive an orientation/training session to review the reading material, answer questions, and practice handling a couple of telephone calls using role playing or sample calls.
3. Observe an experienced telephone care provider handling phone calls for at least 8 hours.

4. Be closely supervised during the first 2 shifts doing telephone care.
5. Have at least 10% of calls reviewed in the first several shifts.

In addition to these steps, each practice should define its own telephone care performance standards. Following are sample performance standards used in primary care practices or medical call centers:

- Documentation—100% of calls for triage and advice or health education are documented.
  - All calls are documented on telephone care documentation forms.
  - Documentation occurs while the provider is speaking to the caller.
- Guidelines—Guidelines are used 100% of the time for telephone triage and advice calls.
  - When a guideline is not available for the presenting problem, advice is obtained from a physician or mid-level practitioner.
  - Guidelines are selected and used in the manner described during training.
- The format and sequence of elements of the model call are followed for each call.
- On average, after the first 3 months on the job, the telephone care provider meets the target call duration (and each call element meets its target duration).
- Callback time—Callback time is within acceptable limits given call volumes and the usual response time in the community.
- Care provider overrides—No more than 5% of the time.
- Caller satisfaction rate—95% satisfactory on survey.
- Complaint rate—Fewer than 1% of callers complain about the provider.
- Attend 75% of telephone care meetings.
- When serious or unusual symptoms are handled, provider will make a follow-up call to determine the outcome.
- Calculate 100% of dosages of over-the-counter medications without error.
- Referral rate—Rate at which patients are referred to be seen in the office or emergency department.
  - In a system with a high level of managed care patients, the rate should be 30% or less after hours.
  - In a capitated environment, the rate should be 50% or less during office hours.
  - In a fee-for-service environment, you may not be interested in tracking referral rate.
- Read and sign *Telephone Care Policy and Procedure Book* every 6 months—100%.
- Arrange for the telephone care manager, or her designee, to observe at least 5 calls at the expected intervals every 6 months for evaluation and feedback. An average rating on the Telephone Care Evaluation Form will be greater than 2.5.

You will, of course, want to develop your own practice telephone care performance standards to promote specific practice goals.

Evaluating Performance

Because there are dual objectives in the performance evaluation process (improvement of skills and determination of retention and salary increases), evaluations should be done by the head nurse or telephone care manager. The focus should be to help the telephone care provider recognize skills that need improvement. The best evaluator is someone who is good at telephone care and teaching and who directly supervises the individual being evaluated.

Evaluations are time consuming, so they should be done at the most effective times in the skill development process. During the initial training period, the trainer will use performance standards to continuously evaluate and give feedback. Formal evaluation may occur at the end of 1 month, 3 months, 6 months, and 1 year. Then, if all is going well, evaluations can be scheduled on a semiannual or annual basis. The evaluation of a telephone care provider can include

- Observation and evaluation of 5 to 10 calls
- Review of the documentation for 10 to 20 calls
- Review of available caller satisfaction data (Chapter 11)
- Review of caller complaints (chapters 12 and 14)
- Review of outcome data (Chapter 14)
- Input from physicians in practice

Assessment of 5 to 10 Calls

The evaluator should directly observe the telephone care provider manage 5 to 10 telephone triage and advice calls and then rate the calls using a call evaluation form like the sample at the end of this chapter. When evaluating performance, it is important to maintain the perspective that the quality of the call is more important than meeting the target times for each component. Adapt the call evaluation form to the performance standards you develop for your practice.

Telephone Documentation Review

The evaluator also should review the logs for 10 to 20 calls to check the adequacy of documentation and apparent adequacy of care, using a form like the sample at the end of this chapter. This also can be done as a peer-review process, in which the telephone care providers review each other's logs using a form like the sample at the end of this chapter. (See also Chapter 14.)

Caller Satisfaction

Caller satisfaction standards for the successful call (Chapter 11) should be incorporated into the performance standards for all office staff members who are involved in telephone care. Caller satisfaction can be assessed using written surveys distributed at office visits or by asking front desk staff to call randomly selected previous callers within a couple of days of their call to the practice and ask a small number of simple questions.

1. Were your questions answered?
2. Were you satisfied with the advice you were given?
3. Was the call handled in a friendly, professional manner?
4. Do you have any suggestions?

Satisfaction surveys can be done during low-volume times of the year and are an important part of maintaining quality of care and patient satisfaction. The survey results can be included in the performance evaluations.

Complaint File

Records of all complaints about telephone care should be kept in a telephone care complaint file. (See chapters 12 and 14.) The provider's complaint rate can be evaluated by (1) dividing the number of complaints about the provider by the number of calls handled by the provider or (2) dividing the number of complaints about the provider by the number of hours worked by the provider providing telephone care. This allows you to compare the complaint rates among telephone care providers.

Outcome Data

Outcome data for telephone care are difficult to obtain in a busy practice. At a minimum, a telephone outcome file can be kept (described in Chapter 14). Keep in the outcome file any information you have collected on outcomes using the outcome log or just informal notes placed in the outcome file by providers in the practice. (See Chapter 14.) Review the lessons learned from the outcome file with the provider.

Periodic Audits

Telephone care audits are an important part of quality improvement and continuing education. (See Chapter 14.) The data obtained can be incorporated into performance evaluations when poor compliance with documentation or guideline usage is identified.

Self-evaluation

Self-evaluation also can improve performance. During the first several months on the job, the telephone care provider can be encouraged to keep the Telephone Care Call Evaluation Form and Telephone Care Documentation Evaluation Form available during calls as a reminder of the performance standards for calls. Telephone care providers also can fill out their own performance evaluation prior to the annual evaluation process and then discuss with the evaluator any significant difference of opinion.

Another approach is for the telephone care provider to regularly observe the response of callers to her actions. Each provider should notice if callers tend to

- Seem argumentative or upset
- Call back with additional questions
- Complain at a higher rate than for other telephone care providers
- Seem uncomfortable with advice

If a provider notices any of these tendencies in her callers, she should ask the telephone care manager to observe her calls in an effort to identify potential causes for these behaviors.

Sample Evaluation Forms

Following are 3 sample evaluation forms. The Telephone Care Call Evaluation Form can be used by the evaluator who observes the provider during 5 to 10 calls. The Telephone Care Documentation Evaluation Form can be used by the evaluator in reviewing documentation. The Telephone Care Provider Evaluation Form can be used by the evaluator to summarize the overall telephone care performance of the provider. These forms can be adapted to your own practice performance standards. Also, these standards and evaluation forms can be incorporated into the evaluation process and forms you may use to evaluate the other roles that the telephone care provider has in the practice.

Final Note

This chapter describes what will appear to be an ambitious performance evaluation process. Try to determine what elements you feel you can actually maintain over the long term and implement those at first. You can always add more later.

TELEPHONE CARE CALL EVALUATION FORM					
Name of Telephone Care Provider_____					
Date_____					
Evaluator_____					
Ratings: 4=excellent 3=good 2=adequate 1=poor 0=not done N/A=not required in call					
	Call #1	Call #2	Call #3	Call #4	Call #5
Greeting appropriate, introduced self					
Verified demographic information					
Actively listened while identifying the presenting problem					
Directed remainder of call					
Assessed onset, duration, severity of symptoms					
Identified chronic problems, chronic medications, allergies					
Selected appropriate guideline					
Used guideline correctly					
Selected appropriate disposition					
Override appropriate					
Advice simple, understandable					
Gave appropriate advice					
Gave callback instructions					
Assessed caller understanding					
Assessed caller comfort					
Professional demeanor					
Was pleasant and respectful to caller					
Was time-efficient for each component					
Documented while speaking with caller					
Appropriate documentation					
Over-the-counter medications calculated correctly					
Actual time of call					

Adapted with permission from evaluation form used in the After-Hours Care Program (pediatric call center) at The Children's Hospital, Denver, CO.

TELEPHONE CARE DOCUMENTATION EVALUATION FORM			

Provider _____ Date _____

Reviewed by _____ Date _____

Information	Absent	Incomplete	Not Applicable
Patient name			
Date of call			
Time			
Gender			
Age			
Caller			
Phone			
Primary care physician			
Chronic disease			
Medications			
Allergies			
Activity level, appearance			
Presenting problem			
Symptoms			
Guideline(s) used			
Disposition			
Care advice			
Callback instructions			
Override and reason			
Caller understanding			
Caller agreement			

TELEPHONE CARE DOCUMENTATION EVALUATION FORM (continued)			
Information	**Absent**	**Incomplete**	**Not Applicable**
Medication (if prescribed)			
Prescription name			
Weight			
Medication allergies			
Pharmacy number			
No calculation errors			
No spelling errors			
Signature			
Total			

Comments:

Adapted with permission from evaluation form used in the call center at Alaska Children's Hospital, Anchorage.

TELEPHONE CARE PROVIDER EVALUATION FORM			
Name of Telephone Care Provider_____			
Date_____			
Evaluator_____			
Ratings: 4=excellent 3=good 2=adequate 1=poor 0=not done N/A=not required in call			
	Rating	**Comments**	**Plan**
Attend quality assurance sessions—75%			
Read and sign *Telephone Care Policy and Procedure Book* every 6 months—100%			
Complaint rate—<1%			
Caller satisfaction rate—95%			
Overall call performance—5 calls			
Specific skills			
Greeting appropriate, introduced self			
Verify demographic information			
Active listening			
Ability to direct the call			
Symptom assessment (onset, duration, severity)			
Identify chronic problems, medications, allergies			
Select appropriate guideline			
Use guidelines correctly			
Select appropriate disposition			
Override appropriate (rate—<5%)			
Advice simple, understandable			
Appropriate advice			
Callback instructions			
Assessment of caller understanding			
Assessment of caller comfort			
Professional demeanor			

TELEPHONE CARE PROVIDER EVALUATION FORM (continued)			
	Rating	**Comments**	**Plan**
Pleasant and respectful to caller			
Time-efficient (call time)			
Document while speaking with caller			
Appropriate documentation			
Over-the-counter medications calculated correctly			
Documentation rate—100%			
Uses guidelines appropriately—100%			
Consults physician appropriately			
Target call duration met?			
Provider overrides <5%			
Caller overrides <5%			
Overall performance			

Adapted with permission from evaluation form used in the After-Hours Care Program (pediatric call center) at The Children's Hospital, Denver, CO.

Chapter 8

Job Descriptions

Job descriptions have the following 3 objectives:

1. Describe the position for prospective employees during recruitment.
2. Define the responsibilities and performance standards to be used in the telephone care provider evaluation process.
3. Define responsibilities and performance standards to support the program evaluation and quality improvement (QI) processes.

The more detailed and objective the job description, the more effectively these objectives can be met. Job descriptions may include the following information:

- Required credentials
- The number of hours to be worked and times of day or night
- Previous experience required (or desired)
- The training required within the practice including expectations for reading
- Requirements for attendance at and participation in telephone care QI and education meetings
- The usual duties during a normal shift (including the model call)
- Care (Chapter 7) and service (Chapter 11) standards (The performance evaluation form can be attached to the job description.)

Sample Job Description

The sample job description offered on the next page includes details that may not fit the needs of your practice or your expectations for every staff member in your practice. Adapt it to your needs and expectations and incorporate it into the job descriptions of all employees who take part in telephone care, even if it is only a small portion of their responsibilities.

Sample Job Description

DENVER FAMILY PRACTICE

Telephone Care Provider

Job Description

Job title: Telephone Care Provider   *Effective date:* _____   *Revision date:* _____

General Description
Use standardized telephone care guidelines to provide telephone triage and advice and health education for callers to the practice.

Experience Required
At least 2 years of primary care practice experience
Good communication skills
Ability to direct the flow of an interview in an efficient manner
Interest in health education
Ability to work independently
Ability to do 2 things at once (multitasking)
Ability to remain calm in emergency situations

Experience Desired
Telephone experience
Ambulatory medical experience

Educational Requirements
Registered nurse degree or licensed practical nurse certification and current state nursing license or equivalent family practice office clinical experience (5 years)
Current basic life support card

Hours to Be Worked

Performance Standards
Correctly use the telephone care guidelines with 100% accuracy.
Document telephone care using documentation forms on 100% of calls.
Attend 75% of the quality improvement sessions and educational sessions.
Read and sign *Telephone Care Policy and Procedure Book* every 6 months.
Read and maintain a working knowledge of the telephone care training materials.
Maintain a complaint rate of <1%.
Maintain a caller satisfaction rate of at least 95%.
Maintain an average call time of 8 minutes or less.
Maintain a pleasant, helpful, professional demeanor.
Be able to calculate medication dosages—100%.
Maintain provider overrides of <5% and patient overrides of <5%.
Use the components of a successful call in proper sequence and within recommended target times.

Adapted with permission from evaluation form used in the After-Hours Care Program (pediatric call center) at The Children's Hospital, Denver, CO.

Chapter 9

Policies and Procedures

Developing policies and procedures is a tedious step and is tempting to avoid. However, there are scores of uncommon, unexpected, and challenging situations and problems related to telephone care that can arise in a family practice for which there are no telephone care guidelines available. While telephone care guidelines provide clinical guidance for symptoms or clinical problems, policies address the nonclinical aspects of telephone encounters. For example, what do you do if a patient who is hearing impaired is trying to reach your office, or a patient who does not speak English calls, or a patient's uncle says he has legal guardianship of a patient and is seeking confidential information, or the telephone service for the whole office goes out, or an 8-year-old is calling for information on child abuse? It is helpful to have a plan in place to guide practice staff members in handling such situations. Well-developed policies and procedures ensure that practice staff respond to these situations appropriately. It also helps reduce medicolegal liability. Telephone care malpractice case law has made it clear that juries expect physicians' offices to use telephone care guidelines, train the telephone care providers, and have established, written office telephone care policies. They also expect all staff members to review them periodically. Because of these expecta-tions, you should require all employees to read the policies and procedures notebook and to document it in a "policy review record" when they have read it.

The policies and procedures notebook should include

- Table of contents
- Policy review record—a record of each time an employee has reviewed the policies and procedures book
- Policies and procedures

The steps for developing a policies and procedure notebook include

1. Selecting the topics and developing a table of contents (situations or problems)
2. Developing a template (or format) for writing the policies
3. Developing the specific policy for each topic and entering it into the template
4. Placing the policies in a notebook
5. Identifying a person who will review the policies periodically for updating and new policy development (usually the telephone care manager)

Remember to make the book available to each telephone care provider and require everyone to read the policies periodically (every 6 months).

Selecting Topics and Developing a Table of Contents

The telephone care medical director, telephone care manager, and experienced telephone care providers in the practice should determine the specifics of the telephone care policies. The challenge is to think of possible special situations and then develop a plan prior to the first occurrence. Of course, there will be unanticipated events for which you will not have a policy. Develop a new policy in response to each special situation so you will be prepared when it recurs.

To assist you in developing your own policies and procedures book, included in this chapter are more than 50 of the most common policies and procedures related to telephone care. You can review and adapt them to your practice and community. Then, using our template, you can create others to address those situations not covered in our samples.

The table of contents can list all of the policies either in alphabetical order or by topic categories. It should indicate when the topic was first issued and last revised. Topics may be listed in more than one location to make it easier for the reader to find those topics that might be thought of by more than one title. For example, the policy on what to do when a caller does not speak English might be listed in the table of contents under (1) the specific name of the language, (2) "foreign language," or (3) "translation services."

Template for Policies

It is helpful to develop a standard format (template) for office telephone policies, which is kept in a computer file. Each time you create a new telephone care policy, you can enter it on the template, print it out, and place it in the book (and add the topic to the table of contents). A sample template is presented at the end of this chapter. Each policy should include at least the following components:

- Topic or subject
- Date the policy was issued
- Last date the policy was revised
- The signature of the person who approved the policy (usually a practice physician, head nurse, or telephone care manager)
- The purpose or objective of the policy
- Which personnel within the practice are affected by the policy (who implements it, who needs to read it)
- Background information (educational or potential resources)
- The policy statement itself
- What documentation will be required about the issue

Policy Review Record

The policy review record records on one page the names of the employees of the practice and the documentation for each time each employee reviewed the policy and procedure book. Each time employees review the book, they place their initials and the date in the appropriate column on this page. The page can be organized in a manner similar to Figure 9-1.

Using Policies

It is important to discuss with all staff members the practice philosophy about policies. The policies cannot anticipate all of the potential situations and nuances that can arise. They are guidelines for general situations, but the staff member will still be called on to use judgment. It is crucial that no one ever say, "Our policy is…." Instead, it is important to convey interest in helping the caller. It also is important to establish a policy on what to do when there is no policy. Who has the authority to make decisions about unusual or difficult situations? Does the telephone care provider have the authority to make independent decisions?

Figure 9-1. Sample Telephone Policies and Procedure Review Record

Denver Family Practice, Inc.
Telephone Policies and Procedure Review Record
Your **Initials** and **Date** below indicate you have read and understand the policies.

NAME	Date	Initials	Date	Initials	Date	Initials	Date	Initials	Date	Initials	Date	Initials

Adapted with permission from evaluation form used in the After-Hours Care Program (pediatric call center) at The Children's Hospital, Denver, CO.

Policies for Patients

Some of the policies relate to how you want callers to use your telephone services. These can be shared with patients and caregivers in a variety of ways. See Chapter 13 for ways to make these policies for patients available in your practice. Although the policies and procedures book may cover some of the policies for patients, it is for staff to use in responding to special situations.

Sample Policies

The following table lists more than 50 telephone policy topics that typically arise in family practice. For each topic, some considerations are suggested. The details of the policy will vary from practice to practice, so you must determine the details of the policies for your practice.

Sample Policies

Suggested Topics	Policy Content
Abuse—calls about abuse or neglect (for example, children, elderly, handicapped)	• Obtain details of situation in open-ended fashion. • Determine if there is any immediate danger to anyone. • Some practices will have a policy to establish contact between caller and a Department of Social Services caseworker or hospital social worker. Other practices will have a policy that all of these calls go to a physician. • If you make a referral to social services, always plan a callback to the social worker to determine the disposition and outcome. • Involve physician.
Ambulance companies—calling for an ambulance	• Telephone number. • What information they usually want. • Criteria for deciding to use ambulance company versus 911 system. • Involve physician.
Answering service problems	• Name, phone number(s) of answering service. • What to do for problems connecting to them or for lost calls. • How to handle complaints about answering service. • How to document problems with answering service.
Appointments	• How to schedule patients over the phone. • Differences in different providers' schedules. • What to tell caller. • When to refer call to nurse for triage (red flag list).
Callbacks	• Types of calls that require a callback: when telephone care provider feels uncomfortable, when caller feels uncomfortable, when telephone care guidelines recommend a callback, after a busy signal or no answer call, when the problem is potentially serious, or when the caller is unable to follow the advice given. • Document all callbacks during which the provider speaks to someone, including all the details of a regular call. • If no answer or busy, just document "no contact," including the caller's name, date, and time.

Sample Policies (continued)

Suggested Topics	Policy Content
Calls, no answer or line busy and no answering machine or voice messaging	• Define how many times you expect the telephone care provider to let the phone ring before quitting (10). • How soon to try again (within 15 minutes). • How and where to document. • How many attempts to make (3).
Calls, unidentified answering machine or voice messaging system	• How many attempts (2). • How long before second attempt (immediate). • What short message to leave on the second attempt (telephone care provider's first name only, "calling from" practice name and primary care physician, indicate the caller's name and phone number you are trying to reach, date and time of call, and office phone number). • How soon to try again (within 15 minutes). • How and where to document.
Calls, identified answering machine or voice messaging system	• Not confidential; not reliable. • Need permission from patient to leave clinical, sensitive, or confidential information on answering machine (leave a message to call practice). • Document. • How many attempts (2), how long before second attempt (15 minutes). • What short message to leave on both attempts (telephone care provider's first name only, "calling from" practice name and primary care physician, indicate the caller's name and phone number you are trying to reach, date and time of call, and office phone number), how soon to try again (within 15 minutes). • How and where to document.
Calls, wrong number	• Try again. • If wrong number, check with message taker (or answering service), try to look up number, assess seriousness of call. • How to document.
Calls, cellular phones	• Notify caller that cellular phones are not confidential. • Ask if the caller would prefer to call back on a corded phone.

Sample Policies (continued)

Suggested Topics	Policy Content
Calls—telephone care provider taking calls for the practice from home	<ul><li>Describe what materials should be at home.</li><li>Standards (if different).</li><li>Qualifications (3+ months' experience during office hours).</li><li>Documentation.</li><li>Time frame within which to get documentation to the office and how.</li></ul>
Chart—when chart needs to be pulled for a phone call	<ul><li>Physician speaking with patient, patient seen in office recently, complicated medical history, prescriptions, etc.</li><li>Some offices pull charts on all clinical calls.</li></ul>
Chronic disease—how to do triage for a patient who has a chronic disease when there is no telephone care guideline	<ul><li>If call is for minor acute illness or problem (eg, diarrhea, colds, trauma), and not the chronic disease, patient can be triaged with appropriate guideline as long as the minor illness does not worsen or relate to symptoms of the chronic disease (eg, cancer patients with fever all are seen immediately).</li><li>When there is a guideline about the chronic disease, use it: asthma attack, eye allergies, hay fever, seizures, febrile seizures, blocked tear ducts.</li><li>If symptoms relate to the chronic disease and there is no guideline, the call goes to the primary care physician.</li></ul>
Complaints/concerns— caller registers a complaint	<ul><li>Provide a standard way to respond: "I am sorry that you are upset (unhappy). Please tell me about it so I can discuss it with the appropriate people here in the practice and we will call you back as soon as we can."</li><li>Who should respond on behalf of the practice? (If complaint is clinical, ask a physician to call back. If it is business-related, either the manager or a physician calls back.)</li><li>Document as much detail as you can.</li></ul>
Confidentiality	<ul><li>Information obtained in telephone care should not be shared with anyone except for clinical care/professional reasons.</li><li>Be aware of (and try to avoid) using phone in places where patients or parents unrelated to the call may be able to hear the conversation.</li><li>Be sure that you are talking with a parent or legal guardian.</li></ul>

Sample Policies (continued)

Suggested Topics	Policy Content
Deaf/hearing- or speech-impaired callers	• Provide the name, number, and procedure for accessing a teletype/teletext or telecommunication device for the hearing or speech impaired when the telephone care provider is asked to return a call to a caller who is hearing impaired. There is usually a state-funded relay operator or program. • Document that this system was used.
Difficult calls—caller disagrees with telephone care provider's recommendations	• If caller wants a higher level of care than is recommended, arrange for that higher level of care, unless possibly harmful, in which case have caller speak to physician. • If caller wants lower level of care than is recommended, have caller speak to physician.
Difficult calls—caller unable to understand advice	• Either give these calls to the physician or arrange for the patient to be seen.
Difficult calls—caller not comfortable with disposition	• Offer to have patient seen or for caller to speak with the physician.
Difficult calls—complicated medical or psychosocial issues	• Arrange an appointment or a callback from a physician.
Difficult callers—calls taking 10 minutes or longer to triage by a skilled telephone triage telephone care provider	• Arrange an appointment or a callback from a physician.
Difficult calls—angry about another aspect of practice	• Describe who in the practice responds to various types of complaints. • Arrange for the caller to speak to that person.
Demand—caller demands to speak to physician	• Describe the practice policy, but if caller insists, accommodate demand.

Sample Policies (continued)

Suggested Topics	Policy Content
Documentation—how to document telephone calls	• Define the minimal documentation expected for all calls. • Explain how to use the documentation form and acceptable abbreviations or shortcuts. • Expect documentation on 100% of all clinical calls (health education or triage and advice calls). • Include a sample telephone log sheet filled out in the way that is expected.
Emergency calls	• Tell how to decide whether to direct the caller to 911 or connect directly to a physician. • List problems that require emergent response. (See Table 6-3 in Chapter 6.)
Emergency department (ED)—arranging to have patient seen in ED	• Telephone numbers of EDs commonly used. • Who to speak to. • What information is normally wanted. • Verbal directions to the ED. • Instructions for when the ED should call the office back. • Insurance restrictions on use of the ED. • Include policy on how to respond to call from ED when patient walks in.
Etiquette on the telephone	• Remind telephone care providers about the skills covered in training, including how you prefer them to greet the caller and identify themselves (first name and title) and the practice. • State how you want callers addressed. • Give sample scripts.
Fax machine—malfunction	• Name and telephone number of company to use to fix the machine. • How to notify the company of the malfunction. • Names and numbers of frequent users or entities that may need urgent access to your practice by fax.
Foreign language—caller does not speak English	• Name and telephone number of telephone translation service. • Process for connecting caller, practice, and translation service. • What to say to caller and translation service. • What to document.

Sample Policies (continued)

Suggested Topics	Policy Content
Greeting—standard greeting for reception and nursing staffs	• Describe the preferred greeting. • Give sample scripts.
Guidelines—when there is no guideline for the problem	• What steps to take when the telephone care provider is unable to decide what guideline to use. • Options: Ask the most experienced telephone care provider or a physician. (See Chronic Disease.)
Laboratory test—ordering outpatient laboratory tests	• What tests can be called in by protocol. • Telephone numbers of laboratories, who to speak to, what information they normally want. • Verbal directions to the laboratory. • Instructions for when the laboratory should call the office back. • Insurance restrictions on use of the laboratory.
Minors—calls from minors	• Describe etiquette such as: show respect for the child, listen respectfully to the question or problem. • Pick an age above which you will respond to the patient alone. Below that age, try to contact the parent. • List the conditions for which you will respond to the child/adolescent without contacting the parent. This is a controversial area, so each practice must make its own decisions.
Neglect—calls about abuse or neglect	• See Abuse.
Over-the-counter medications	• See sample policy at the end of this chapter.
Overrides—telephone care provider overrides disposition in guideline	• Telephone care provider may override the telephone care guideline if the telephone care provider feels child is sicker than the disposition acknowledges, parent is not comfortable with disposition or advice, or telephone care provider is not sure of the correct guideline.
Overwhelmed patient or caller—unable to cope with life stresses	• Determine what resources your practice can offer this type of caller. • List criteria for using those resources. • List phone numbers of local resources. • Questions to ask to determine risks to the child. • Telephone care provider should be empathic, patient, and understanding.

Sample Policies (continued)

Suggested Topics	Policy Content
Pay phones—parents calling from pay phones	• Try to respond completely to the call at the time of the call rather than call back.
Physician—when should telephone care provider turn the call over to the physician	• List which kinds of calls should always be referred to the physician (ie, emergencies, sick neonates, complicated medical history, patient insists, calls from other professionals, hospitals).
Physician—how to handle calls from physicians	• In which instances should the practice physician be interrupted and when should a message be taken. • Suggest how to ask for the information to make the decision.
Physician—handling calls when physician is out of the office	• Pager numbers of physicians. • Criteria for when to page physician and when messages can wait until next planned contact with physician. • Determine a length of time that certain messages can wait before physician responds. • When to page again.
Physician—parent asks to speak to physician	• Determine criteria for patients speaking to physician.
Poisonings	• Give the caller the number of the poison control center. • Be sure the caller is able to call the poison control center. • Do follow-up call to be sure the caller was adequately served. • If no poison control center available, use guidelines for common poisoning protocols.
Prescription medications—calling in new prescriptions	• List medications telephone care provider can call in on own (per guideline). • What information to get from patients (weight; allergies; pharmacy name, location, and phone number). • What information to give patient/caller (medication name, dosage, frequency, route, duration and instructions, callback instructions). • What information to give to pharmacy (patient name, birthday, home number, primary care physician name, medication name, dose/concentration, frequency, duration, route, weight, allergies, number of refills). • How to document in chart. • The numbers of the most commonly used pharmacies.

Sample Policies (continued)

Suggested Topics	Policy Content
Prescription medications—calling in prescription refills	• List medication refills telephone care provider can call in on own (per guideline). • What information to get from patients (weight; allergies; pharmacy name, location, and phone number). • What information to give patient/caller (medication name, dosage, frequency, route, duration and instructions, callback instructions). • What information to give to pharmacy (number on the original prescription if filled at that pharmacy, patient name, birthday, home number, primary care physician name, medication name, dose/concentration, frequency, duration, route, weight, allergies, number of refills). • How to document in chart. • The numbers of the most commonly used pharmacies.
Callers who are not related to the patient	• If patient is with them and unable to talk on the phone, handle as if they are the caregiver. If the patient is a competent adult, ask to speak to the patient. If patient is not with them and they are just calling for information about patient, suggest they speak with the patient.
Repeat callers—acute	• Two calls in 24 hours about same problem, offer appointment. • Three calls about the same illness, urge them to have an appointment.
Repeat callers—chronic	• When you notice that a patient is a frequent caller, suggest an appointment. • Make a note in frequent-caller file to discuss at next telephone care meeting.
Suicide—caller is threatening suicide or is family member or caregiver of patient talking of suicide	• Ask for name and telephone number and address where the caller is calling from. • Be calm, patient, and empathetic. • Determine immediate danger, whether to patch 911 onto the call. • Determine if risk to others, whether to call police. • Patch the local suicide line or emergency mental health resource into the call, if available.

Sample Policies (continued)

Suggested Topics	Policy Content
Telephone breakdown or not working (line/set)	• Describe how to determine if it is the phone, the individual line, or all lines into the office. • If it is the phone, have a priority list of acceptable replacements in the office and bring it to the telephone care station. • If it is the line, have a list of alternative locations to move to. • If it is all lines to the office, prioritize the existing calls to see if anyone needs to make a home visit or go to another location to make the calls. • Document times of the shutdown. • List names of companies that hold service contracts on equipment.
Visitor—out-of-town visitor in the home of a patient calling for advice	• Treat as though patient is in the practice, but obtain more details of chronic problems, medications, allergies, and demographics. • Document. • Low threshold to see patient.
Voice messaging systems	See Calls.

Adapted with permission from policies used in the After-Hours Telephone Care Program (pediatric call center) at The Children's Hospital, Denver, CO.

Sample Policy Template

DENVER FAMILY PRACTICE, INC.
TELEPHONE CARE POLICIES

SUBJECT: Standing Orders: Refill Prescription Medications

	DATE ISSUED	2/5/96
APPROVED BY:_____	DATE REVISED	12/07/00

PURPOSE: To provide guidelines for refill prescription medication orders over the telephone

PERSONNEL: Telephone care providers only

GENERAL INFORMATION

All refill prescription medication orders and guidelines have been reviewed and approved by the practice physicians and head telephone care provider. They are consistent with the advice given in the telephone care guidelines. They are consistent with the standards of nursing practice published by the Colorado State Nursing Board.

POLICY STATEMENT

Refill prescription medication policies apply only to patients registered in the practice with an active chart in the file and who have been seen in the past year.

Refill prescriptions may be called in if
- The medication was prescribed within the last year (12 months).
- The prescription is called ONLY to the original pharmacy that filled the prescription, not to a new pharmacy.
- The condition, for which the patient is receiving medications, is not worsening and has no new symptoms.
- If the chronic disease is covered by a protocol, triage the patient before approving the refill (eg, asthma attack).
- Antibiotics.
  - If patient is on a continuous or maintenance antibiotic (eg, ear infection or urinary tract infection given prophylactically once per day), may give a 4-week supply.
  - If antibiotic was spilled, lost, or misplaced (ie, left at child care over the weekend), a refill is allowed for the number of days remaining on the current prescription ONLY.

Refill prescription **MAY NOT** be called in for the following, unless approved by a physician:
- Controlled or restricted substances
- Steroid bursts

If above criteria for refill prescription medications are not met, the telephone care provider should leave a message for the primary care physician to call back.

The telephone care provider will obtain the following information from the caller before ordering a refill prescription medication:
- Patient's weight
- Known allergies

Sample Policy Template (continued)

- Pharmacy name, location, and telephone number
- Prescription number on label
- Physician listed on label
- Medication information read from the prescription label

The telephone care provider instructs the caller on the prescription medication
- Name of medication
- Dosage
- Frequency
- Route
- Length of administration (antibiotics and refills)
- Administration instructions
- Callback instructions

The caller should confirm understanding of instructions.

The telephone care provider provides the following information to the pharmacy:
- Patient's name
- Birth date
- Home telephone number
- Primary care physician name and office number
- Medication name
- Prescription number from label
- Dose with concentration
- Frequency
- Length of administration (ie, antibiotics) or amount to be ordered (eg, Nystatin 60-mL bottle)
- Route (only if other than by mouth)
- Weight of patient (as appropriate for prescription order)
- Allergies (if any)
- No refills

DOCUMENTATION

Refill prescription medication orders should be documented with the following information:
- Pharmacy (of original prescription) name and telephone number. If refill order is to be transferred electronically to another associated pharmacy, include the name and location of both pharmacies.
- Prescription number.
- Physician name (matching the primary care physician).
- Medication name.
- Dosage with concentration.
- Frequency.
- Route.
- Weight of patient.
- Known allergies.
- Care advice and callback instructions given.

Adapted with permission from policy used in the After-Hours Telephone Care Program (pediatric call center) at The Children's Hospital, Denver, CO.

Chapter 10

Supplies, Equipment, and Work Space

Materials and Supplies

Professionals are more effective when the tools of their trade are readily available. Telephone care providers will need a variety of materials and supplies to support their efforts, including

- A dedicated telephone and outgoing telephone line, along with access to at least one other office line. The telephone should have the following functions: automatic redial, transfer, conference call, hold, mute, and speakerphone. Ideally, a "hands-free" headset should be available.
- A supportive, comfortable chair.
- An adjustable footrest for those with back or leg symptoms.
- A set of telephone care guidelines.
- Telephone log sheets.
- A copy of the practice telephone policy book.
- A list of community resources, programs, and educational offerings.
- A list of important phone and fax numbers (ie, pharmacies, emergency departments, physician referral line, ambulance and transport services, poison center, child protective services, public health department, sexual assault resources, and police department).
- Guidelines for scheduling and making appointments in the practice.
- A dosage chart for common over-the-counter (OTC) medications.
- A chart for converting pounds to kilograms and centigrade to fahrenheit.
- A list of normal laboratory values.
- Current references such as
    - *Physicians' Desk Reference* (prescription and OTC).
    - *Merck Manual* or other medication interaction reference.
    - A family medicine textbook.
    - *Harriet Lane Handbook.*
    - Current immunization schedule.
    - A medical dictionary.
    - A breastfeeding guide, including information on medications in human milk and contraindications to breastfeeding.
- Calculator.
- Scratch paper.
- Plenty of pens.

Some of these reference materials are available now online or will be available as time goes by.

The following list of materials will be useful for the reception/scheduling staff and, because the telephone care providers may need to give information like that provided by the front office telephone staff or may make appointments, they will need these supplies, too:

- Instructions for callers about directions to the office or frequently used referral sources
- Access to the office appointment schedule.
- The list of red-flag symptoms or problems that should be turned over to a clinical staff person.
- The answers to common questions about charges and billing.

Work Space

The actual work area has some important requirements.

- Adequate space, including room for a desk, bookshelves, and a comfortable and ergonomically appropriate chair. A "workstation" is ideal.
- Quiet, calm location away from high-traffic areas.
- Enough separation from other activities to allow confidentiality for the callers.
- Close proximity to medical records.

Sharing Space With Scheduling Staff

Larger practices (perhaps 8 physicians or more or when there are multiple offices) can consider locating the scheduling personnel with the telephone care providers away from the front desk. The reception staff at the front desk can do check-in and check-out. The scheduling staff can make telephone appointments, take messages, answer simple telephone questions, pull charts, and help the telephone care providers, all in a quieter, less chaotic environment. By working together with the telephone care provider(s) they can make one another more efficient. By sitting together, they can answer questions for one another and hand calls off to one another in a manner that is more efficient for the caller.

Chapter 11

Caller Satisfaction

Clinical care is an important part of the entire telephone-related experience; however, a variety of other factors also contribute to the caller's satisfaction. Just as a telephone care provider is expected to meet clinical performance standards, she also should understand and meet the caller's service-oriented expectations.

The Successful Call (From the Caller's Perspective)

The first step in improving caller satisfaction is to define the successful call from the standpoint of the caller. There are 3 possible ways to do this: (1) conduct a survey of patients in the practice, (2) informally query a few patients you know well, or (3) have the staff anticipate what callers would want (using their office experience and their own experience as patients). Just as in developing clinical performance standards, the more quantitative you can be, the easier it will be to measure success or failure in meeting your objectives. Consider developing caller satisfaction expectations for the parameters listed in Table 11-1, determining your own specific quantitative objectives for each parameter. These target standards are based on those that a large primary care practice in Denver, CO, set for itself. Each practice will have to determine what is reasonable in its own practice, and expectations may have to be different for winter than for summer.

Quality Improvement Projects (See Chapter 14.)

Periodic quality improvement audits can focus on any of the caller satisfaction expectations. For example, during a low-volume time, someone affiliated with the practice can make mock calls to the practice to measure response times, time on hold, frequency with which greetings and introductions meet standards, and so on. Or you can track certain of these parameters for a period until you are comfortable that you are meeting the standard frequently enough. Your local telephone company has the technology to track certain data for you, such as number of rings until answered and time on hold. The other parameters can be tracked manually in the office. However, what you really want to know is the perception of the caller. This is best determined with a caller satisfaction survey.

Caller Satisfaction Survey

The objective of a caller satisfaction survey is to assess how well the practice meets its caller satisfaction standards (the successful call from the caller's perspective). There are several ways to accomplish this.

1. Written survey mailed to patients
2. Written survey handed out at office visits
3. Telephone survey of recent callers to the practice, conducted during low-volume times by the reception staff

Option 1 is expensive and tends to yield a low response rate. Option 2 may be the simplest, but option 3 will obtain the best response rate. The questions on the written questionnaire or telephone survey should include the following:

1. Was your call answered in a timely manner?
2. Did our staff respond in a professional, pleasant, friendly manner?
3. Did our staff listen well to you?
4. Did we answer your question or concern to your satisfaction?
5. What suggestions for improvement do you have for us?

If you need to shorten the survey, at least include a question about suggestions because that usually is the best source of ideas for improvement.

The overall results of the survey should be shared with the group to initiate a discussion of what changes are needed. Caller satisfaction standards can be included in all of the standards of performance for all telephone care providers. Results of the caller satisfaction survey for individuals can be used in performance evaluations.

Your Telephone System

Few voices can be friendly or helpful enough to the caller who has been on hold for 15 minutes. Long call holds can result in longer calls and more callers being on hold longer. When speaking to a caller who is frustrated because of a long hold time, expect the caller to need time to complain, refocus, be reassured, and regain his or her confidence. All of this causes successive callers to experience additional delays—a vicious cycle from which it may be difficult to recover.

Systems that allow callers to leave voice mail may be helpful, but are only useful if messages are listened to and an appropriate response is provided in a timely manner. It is very important when using a voice mail system to change outgoing messages to inform people about times when calls will go unanswered for unusually long periods.

Equally important are the reliability of your system and its ease of use to your staff and callers. The ability of your system to provide data on calls is an important tool for improving caller satisfaction. Reports on the number of calls received, how long callers are on hold, the number of calls unanswered after a reasonable time, and the average length of calls are examples of useful management tools. This information can be helpful in planning for satisfaction with phone management. These reports should be reviewed on a regular basis and used when considering staffing practices, patient enrollment, patient retention, efficiency, and productivity. On a periodic basis, providers who usually call their office on a "back line" should call using the same system the patients use. This can help in understanding the pitfalls patients could face when calling. After-hours call management is equally important. The entire telephone system should be assessed periodically to ensure that callers receive the level of service from your office that you intend for them.

Table 11-1 **Sample Caller Satisfaction Expectations for the Successful Call**	
Parameter	**Standard**
Number of rings before call answered	2
Friendly greeting, "smile over the phone"	100%
Standard office greeting used	100%
Office staff introduces self at beginning of call	100%
Maximum length of time on hold	20 seconds
If there is an automated attendant, ● Maximum length ● Maximum number of levels of options ● Ability to opt to speak to a person	 20 seconds 5 Within 20 seconds
No contact calls to practice ("hang-ups")	<2%
If unable to respond when caller calls in, the maximum wait time for a callback ● Emergency ● Urgent ● Nonurgent	 Immediate 10 minutes 60 minutes
Complaint rate	<1%
Caller will say staff was professional, friendly, organized	99%
Caller will say staff answered questions to his or her satisfaction	>95%

Chapter 12

Complaint Resolution

A complaint is an opportunity. Complaints can

1. Enable the telephone care provider to learn something new to improve care and service.
2. Help evaluate the performance of the telephone care provider.
3. Enable the improvement of the quality of telephone care in the practice as a whole.
4. Improve the relationship between the practice and caller who is complaining.
5. Lead to the fair resolution of a problem or dispute.

The most helpful attitude for individuals, and for the practice as a whole, is to consider a complaint as an opportunity to learn and improve clinical care and service. When an honest attempt is made to accomplish the first 4 objectives, then objective 5 is usually accomplished as well.

Educating the Telephone Care Provider

There is something to learn from every complaint. Sharing the complaint with the telephone care provider as soon as is convenient allows the supervisor to hear the provider's side and develop a more balanced perspective about the complaint. The supervisor can establish a helpful atmosphere by asking the provider what she thinks can be learned from the complaint. It is helpful to ask the provider how she thinks this feedback could and should affect the management of calls in the future, both for herself and for all telephone care providers in the practice. If the supervisor feels there are additional learning points, those can be shared and discussed.

Evaluating Each Telephone Care Provider

Each telephone care provider's evaluation should include a review of all complaints and concerns about calls handled by her, including learning points and constructive suggestions. A completed caller complaint form (see sample at the end of this chapter) should be included in the performance evaluation file for the telephone care provider. The focus during the yearly performance evaluation should be on helping the provider improve clinical care and service by reviewing these complaints.

Quality Improvement

Quality improvement for care and service is described in Chapter 14. At regularly scheduled telephone care meetings, the group can review in an anonymous fashion the complaints that have been received since the last meeting. The group can discuss how to handle those calls to reduce the likelihood of complaints. Often these are difficult calls or callers, from which other providers can learn.

Improving the Relationship With the Caller

The relationship between the caller and practice nearly always improves when the caller recognizes that the practice views the complaint as an opportunity to learn and improve.

The return call to the caller who complained usually should come from the telephone care manager, practice manager, or patient's primary care physician. The following format for handling complaints is usually successful:

First Call
1. "Hello, this is _____, the head nurse from Denver Family Practice. I am calling in response to the concern you expressed about a recent call to our practice. Could you please fill me in?"
2. Active listening; asking for clarification so you will understand their point of view.
3. Show you understand the caller's feelings. "I can see that you are very upset." "You were very worried about your child." "You must have been frustrated."
4. Apologize that the caller had a bad experience. "I am sorry that the call did not go as you had hoped. We want to meet your needs."
5. Explain that the practice views complaints as an opportunity to learn and improve.
6. Explain that you want to talk to the telephone care provider and go over the complaint.
7. In most instances, plan to call the person back to report the outcome.
8. Talk to the telephone care provider between calls.
9. Look for a new policy or policy change that may be needed. Understand what the telephone care provider, and the others, could learn from the complaint.
10. Decide on a fair resolution to the complaint.

Second Call
1. Call the person back. Describe what you, the telephone care provider, or the practice learned.
2. Describe any action planned.
3. Apologize if appropriate.
4. Thank the caller for bringing this to your attention.

Remember
- Listen respectfully and nonjudgmentally and take the complaint seriously.
- Be understanding of the caller's feelings.
- If the caller has experienced financial loss, be sure to check with the liability insurer before deciding on any restitution.
- Minimize any further inconvenience for the caller.
- Be sure the caller knows that people have discussed the complaint and looked for what can be learned from it.
- Reassure the caller that appropriate changes will be made.
- Thank the caller for communicating with you.

Document both the calls and the discussion with the telephone care provider briefly, and keep it in a file as long as the provider is in the practice or any poor outcome or litigation remains possible, whichever is longer. If there is a chance of litigation, discuss with the appropriate practice owners/management and then with the professional liability insurance representative.

Resolution will come by following the 5 steps and making sure that you treat the complainant with respect and fairness. Remember: One bad experience for a patient usually will be retold to 10 other people.

COMPLAINT RESOLUTION FORM

Name of Caller: _____   Date: _____

Telephone Number: _____   Time: _____

Name of Telephone Care Provider:

Complaint by Caller About:

Service: _____

_____

_____

Clinical Care: _____

_____

_____

Telephone Care Provider's Version: _____

_____

_____

Learning Points for Telephone Care Provider: _____

_____

_____

Performance Evaluation: _____

_____

_____

Resolution: _____

_____

_____

Chapter 13

Educating Callers

If you can successfully educate callers about how to appropriately and efficiently use the telephone to access your practice, you will reduce unnecessary calls, improve office efficiency, reduce expenses, improve quality of telephone care, and reduce medicolegal risk. To educate patients about your telephone care policies, create an organized, succinct summary of what you want patients to know about how to access your office by phone. Then you can provide this summary to all patients in the practice using a

- Handout at health maintenance visits or first-time appointments
- Section in the practice's patient information handout
- Brief summary on the telephone message that callers hear while on hold
- Section on your practice Web site

Office Policy for Patients

The office telephone policy for patients might include the following components:

- Rationale and purpose of telephone triage and advice.
- Health information resources.
  - Books you recommend.
  - Handouts.
  - Practice booklet.
  - Practice Web site.
  - Health information lines available in the community.
- When and what number to call.
  - For illness advice.
  - For illness appointment.
  - For emergencies.
  - For poisonings.
  - For health maintenance questions.
  - For prescription refills.
  - Nights, weekends, holidays.
- Information to have available for the call.
  - Medical history.
  - Onset/duration/severity.
  - Why calling now.
  - Weight/temperature.
  - Hydration: urine output, oral intake.
  - Pharmacy phone number.
  - Insurance information.

- How to present information.
  - State if it is an emergency.
  - Start with the symptom most concerned about, omit extraneous information.
- How to use advice.
  - Write down instructions.
  - Tell the telephone care provider if there are any barriers to care.
- How and when to use the fax instead of phone.
- A reminder to unblock the telephone for a callback.

The office telephone policy for patients at the end of this chapter is a sample. Almost every practice differs in the way it prefers to handle telephone calls, so you will have to adapt the sample to meet the specific needs and expectations of your practice.

SAMPLE TELEPHONE POLICY STATEMENT FOR PATIENTS

Emergency Calls (Day or Night)
- Call 911 (emergency medical services) for any life-threatening emergencies (eg, severe difficulty breathing, severe choking, knocked unconscious, severe chest pain, excessive bleeding).
- Our practice is always available for minor emergencies (eg, dehydration, difficulty breathing, suturing, fractures).
- When you call in, always state clearly, "This is an emergency." Do not let the answering service or office staff put you on hold.
- Poisoning: The Poison Control Center can be reached by calling _____.

Calls About Illness During Office Hours
We see patients with illnesses by appointment only. Our office hours are:
weekdays _____ to _____, Saturday _____ to _____, and Sunday_____ to _____.

The telephone nurse is available to take your calls _____ minutes before the office opens. If you or a family member is sick and you want him or her seen, call ahead for an appointment so you will not have to wait. Try to call us about your illness during the early morning office hours. All medical calls are screened by a telephone nurse who has been specially trained to make decisions on which patients need to be seen and how to provide home care for those who do not need to be seen. If the telephone nurse cannot help you, you will be asked to come in or have your physician call you back. If the office staff is busy and can only take a message, ask for an approximate callback time. While waiting for a callback, try to keep your line open. If your call is not returned within 60 minutes after the predicted callback time, call again. In general, we try to return calls within 15 minutes. Keep in mind that Monday mornings are the busiest time.

Working Patients and Parents
We keep appointments open during the last hour of the day for adults or children who need to be seen after work, school, or child care. Be certain your baby-sitter or child care center understands they should call you before 3:00 pm if your child becomes ill. If you think your child may need to be seen today, please call before our office closes.

(continued on next page)

SAMPLE TELEPHONE POLICY STATEMENT FOR PATIENTS, *continued*

Prescription Refills
We refill prescriptions only during office hours. We need your chart handy to check on dosages and the disease status. Plan ahead so you do not run out of important medicines. Always have the phone number of your pharmacy available before you call the office.

Nighttime (After-Hours) Calls
After office hours, calls should be made only for emergencies or urgent problems that cannot wait until morning. At night our line needs to be kept open for these purposes. Calls about mild illnesses usually can wait until the next morning. During these hours your calls will be received by an answering service and transferred to your physician or the telephone nurse who is covering your physician's calls. They will usually return your call within 15 to 30 minutes. If you do not receive a return call within 1 hour in a nonemergency situation, please call again.

Weekend and Holiday Calls
If you or a family member becomes ill or injured, call your physician's answering service. Try to call before noon so we can plan the day. Again, calls after 5:00 pm should be limited to those about emergencies or other urgent problems that cannot wait until morning.

Information Before Calling
Please know the following (except in emergencies):

- The main symptoms.
- If you have a chronic disease or health problem, be sure to mention it.
- Your temperature if you are sick.
- Your approximate weight (for calculating drug dosage).
- The names and dosages of any medicines you are taking.
- Your pharmacy's telephone number.
- Your questions written down.
- Finally, have a pencil and paper handy to take down instructions and, if you are calling about an ill family member, have the family member nearby, in case something needs to be checked.

This policy statement was developed by Barton D. Schmitt, MD. Reprinted with permission.

Chapter 14

Quality Improvement and Ongoing Telephone Care Education

In 1998 the Institute of Medicine published its now famous report, "To Err Is Human," and in 2001 it published a second report, "Crossing the Quality Chasm." Both publications documented that a substantial number of errors occur in all areas of medical practice and urged all physicians to objectively analyze errors and sources of errors to improve the quality of care. In a family practice, quality improvement (QI) involves evaluating clinical processes, identifying problems, determining the causes, correcting them, and then reevaluating them at a later time. Assessing quality in a family practice can be difficult because of the lack of time, resources, and support.

The Quality Improvement Process
The QI process can be used to (1) evaluate and improve selected elements of your telephone care system or (2) identify and solve specific problems. The QI process involves 6 steps. When evaluating an element of telephone care

1. Select a performance parameter to evaluate and improve.
2. Observe and measure the performance parameter (ideally measure how well you meet a standard you have set).
3. Use the observations and measurements to identify specific deficiencies you want to change.
4. Design and implement a plan to improve the deficiencies, then enact the plan.
5. Observe and measure performance after the plan is enacted and adapt the plan as needed.
6. Measure performance at a later time to see if the improvement has been maintained.

For example, you might decide to evaluate clinical call duration. Measure call duration on all calls for a week. Compare it with your standard (expected average call duration). If the average for the group is long, make additional observations (eg, call durations for individuals, durations for the components of calls). Perhaps you find that most telephone care providers are spending too much time actively listening and taking the initial history. As a group, discuss ways to reduce the duration of this clinical call component and develop a plan for improving call duration. Implement the plan. Remeasure a couple of weeks later and modify the plan if needed. Then plan to remeasure again in a couple of months.

When you already have a problem in mind, the steps are

1. Select the problem.
2. Observe (measure) the problem to identify causes.
3. Articulate the specific deficiencies you want to change and observe or measure them.
4. Design and implement a plan.
5. Observe and measure the problem again relatively soon.
6. Reevaluate it later.

Quality improvement in telephone triage may be best achieved by incorporating it into the evaluation and improvement of the whole continuum of the care provided by the practice. In other words, develop a QI system for the practice as a whole; telephone care QI can be one component of that QI system.

In most practices, nursing staff rotate between telephone triage duties and other patient care on a regular basis. The staff should be very actively involved in quality assessment and QI in all areas. When staff members are involved in a QI process, they can better identify problems, have better insight into the causes of the problems, and are much more motivated to participate in sustained efforts to improve care.

Problem Identification

It is important to have an organized approach for identifying problems. Three approaches include (1) maintaining files of complaint calls, difficult calls, and calls with poor outcomes; (2) using caller satisfaction surveys; and (3) conducting audits of selected issues and parameters. In addition, office staff also may be able to identify a problem that they wish to explore in detail.

Complaint File

Complaint resolution is discussed in Chapter 12. "Every complaint is a gift" and can be an excellent stimulus for improving care. All complaints about telephone care should be kept in a file for QI as well as individual performance evaluation (Chapter 7). Complaints can be discussed at each telephone care meeting in an anonymous fashion, emphasizing what can be learned by the group from the complaint. If the problem is of significant magnitude and/or frequency, the group may decide to study it further and implement changes in policies or procedures.

Difficult or Problem Call File

Each time a telephone care provider handles a call that involves an issue or problem not previously handled, a brief summary should be placed in a file for review at a telephone care meeting. The staff can decide whether to evaluate the problem using the QI process.

Outcomes File

Later in this chapter, methods for determining outcomes of calls are described. When a call with a poor outcome is identified, it can be placed in a file for later review at a telephone care meeting. During the review, problems in the telephone care process may be identified.

Caller Satisfaction Survey

Sometimes health plans conduct surveys and share practice-specific data with individual practices. If these data are available, be sure to review them and share the data relevant to telephone care with the telephone care providers. If these types of data are not available, consider conducting a brief telephone survey of previous callers during low-call volume times (Chapter 11). Staff can call randomly selected previous callers a couple of days after they have called the practice for telephone care to ask a few simple questions.

1. Was your call answered in a timely manner?
2. Did our staff respond in a professional, pleasant, friendly manner?

3. Did our staff listen well to you?

4. Did we answer your question or concern to your satisfaction?

5. What suggestions for improvement do you have for us?

The most useful information can come from question 5. This information, especially the suggestions, can be shared in an anonymous fashion at a telephone care meeting.

Audits

An audit can be used to evaluate elements of a telephone care program and identify problems that deserve further assessment (more auditing), as described under the Quality Improvement Process section. Each of the elements of the model triage and advice call lends itself to being audited, then discussed to determine the best way to provide that component in a high-quality and efficient manner. Potential topics for audit include call times, guideline selection, consistency of documentation, frequency of dispositions of calls, and frequency of and reasons for overrides (deviations from guidelines) by either the patient or telephone care provider.

Observe/Measure the Problem or Performance Parameter

Clearly define the problem or parameter you wish to observe and measure. Think of ways to measure these parameters quantitatively, if possible. It is difficult enough to collect all of the information and track the data that health plans require let alone trying to collect more information, so it is important to only collect information that you will use and to use the information that you collect. Following are suggestions for ways to collect information on telephone care performance parameters and problems. We have tried not to recommend anything that is too time-consuming or expensive. Each practice can select a few things to do among these options.

We are all aware of the Hawthorne effect. When human activities are simply observed, the process of observing the activity creates changes. In addition to collecting useful information about the issue and identifying areas needing improvement, the audit serves to increase the level of awareness about the issue. By evaluating an action or process, the evaluator usually develops a deeper understanding and appreciation of the issue.

Audits are a very effective tool for evaluating group performance and changing it. At one telephone care meeting you can plan the audit. The audit can be conducted by the telephone care providers between meetings, and the results can be discussed at the next meeting. When first auditing a new topic, the audit duration should be short—a week or two. The results should be shared immediately and any new planning and changes in implementation discussed soon after. Then a new, longer duration audit can be conducted. This allows the group to quickly recognize the obvious problems, adjust the plan to handle them early in the process, and then use the longer audit to fine-tune the issues. Audits often lead to policy changes. Audits also are a form of continuing education.

Auditing Performance Standards

Auditing performance standards (Chapter 7) allows you to evaluate how well you are routinely implementing your basic telephone care program (your baseline). When the telephone care provider group decides to audit a certain topic, attention should be focused on that one issue. To be useful, the data should be gathered in a standardized manner on specially developed forms. It is important that everyone who will collect data agree on how to collect and record the data in a uniform way. It is helpful to have someone observe each data collector to be sure everyone is doing it the same way. The following audits have proven useful in family practices and warrant your consideration.

Documentation

To audit telephone care documentation, each telephone care provider can be given the logs for 10 to 20 randomly selected clinical calls handled by other providers to review. Using the Telephone Care Documentation Evaluation Form (Chapter 7), each provider determines whether each log entry meets practice standards. Providers note whether everything is documented, was legible, was understandable, met criteria for brevity, and so on. The process of deciding what to audit on the telephone logs serves to initiate the discussion of what the ideal documentation should look like in your office. The process of auditing logs helps the provider develop a deeper understanding and appreciation of the need for complete documentation. The audit encourages better overall compliance. Most importantly, the discussion will lead to new and better policies on documentation.

Call Times

Keep track of the duration of all calls (and perhaps the duration of selected components of the call, like the greeting, active-listening portion of the call, guideline questions, advice, or closure) for a 1- or 2-week period. Simply observing call times usually reduces call duration. This also may provide information that may enable the improvement of telephone care staffing in the practice. The ensuing discussion can lead to changes in the model call, target call duration, or target times for certain elements of the call.

Patient Overrides

You can design a brief survey for the telephone care providers to administer to those callers who do not feel comfortable with or do not want to follow the advice they are given. The questions should attempt to understand why patients in your practice override the disposition or advice. The telephone care provider might say, "Help me understand what you are thinking or feeling about the advice." As the provider listens to the answer, she can decide whether the override is a matter of convenience, patient anxiety, disagreement with the clinical decision making, or other issues. The results can lead to a discussion of how best to respond to patient overrides and perhaps to the development of new policies.

Telephone Care Provider Overrides

Keep track of all telephone care provider overrides for a month, noting the reason for the override and outcome for the patient. As you recognize reasons, patterns, and habits, the ensuing discussion may lead to new policies and help some providers adapt their styles.

Guideline Selection Audit

An audit of symptom guideline selection can be very instructive. An audit can be performed by gathering data on all calls performed over a defined period. Over that period, the proportions of guidelines selected by each provider should be similar. If there are significant differences among providers in how often they use various guidelines, the providers can discuss their decision-making process and perhaps come to a consensus.

Telephone Care Disposition Audits

An audit can be performed periodically to determine if there are major differences in the dispositions reached among providers. The auditor should focus on what guideline was used and the disposition reached. The relative proportion of dispositions recommended by providers should be similar for the same guidelines. If a particular nurse has excessive "home care" dispositions or another has an increased number of "see immediately" dispositions, this may indicate over-referral or under-referral, and a detailed review of triage techniques may be indicated.

Auditing Specific Problems

Problems that have been previously identified through complaint, poor outcomes, or earlier audits can be observed in the same way as performance parameters. The audit can determine how often the problem occurs, what factors appear to contribute to its occurrence, and the effect on the caller or patient. During the audit, telephone care providers and callers might be asked for their opinion on possible solutions.

Identify and Carefully Consider the Deficiencies in the Process of Care That Contribute to Poor Performance

Audits can be useful tools for measuring baseline performance and identifying problems. However, staff and physician leaders need to recognize that it is often difficult to identify why problems occur. Recognizing the underlying reasons requires considerable time and thought. The team needs to brainstorm about the likely sources of the problem.

This root cause analysis is very helpful when developing meaningful strategies to improve performance. An example in telephone triage could be to evaluate why the practice has a high number of repeat calls about fever in children. On first glance, it may be postulated that telephone care providers do not inform parents about when to call back. More detailed evaluation may reveal that repeat calls occurred because of persistence of fever. Further evaluation may reveal that the practice does not routinely provide parents with optimal dosages for antipyretics. It also may be realized that the care advice emphasizing effectiveness of antipyretics (lowering fever by an average of 2°F) is not routinely shared in an effort by the staff to reduce call time. A final analysis also may reveal that the practice may be unintentionally creating fear in parents about fever during office visits. The time spent by staff to determine causes of problems is critical to QI.

Designing and Implementing a Plan to Improve Performance

This often is the most stimulating and rewarding task in QI. When office staff are involved in planning, they usually better understand the value of doing things differently and become highly vested in the success of the plan. It is important to make realistic changes that are easy to implement. It also is important to make sure that improvements in performance can be easily monitored and evaluated.

Measuring Performance After an Intervention and at a More Distant Time

The best way to demonstrate improvement is to use the same data gathering tools that were used in the initial evaluation phase. Evaluate the new plan soon after it is implemented and make the evaluation period relatively brief (a few days or weeks) to collect information needed to adapt the plan, if necessary.

It is important to again think of the Hawthorne effect. Positive changes may diminish after the period of observation and special focus. This is especially true when the office staff has been very involved in designing the intervention. It is, therefore, imperative to measure performance again at a more distant time to ensure that the improvement in performance persists. Although a QI exercise usually is effective, some interventions may be truly ineffective, and the team may need to remain open, reevaluate the problem, and reconsider the causes of the problem and the intervention designed.

Continuing Education

Outcomes

The most effective teacher is experience. So it is helpful for the telephone care provider to be allowed time to actually see some patients she has advised to come in for an appointment, especially those who sounded sicker than usual over the phone. It also is useful for the telephone care providers to take a look at charts to learn more details about the patients referred for care, including the diagnosis. The physicians or mid-level practitioners who see the patients also can provide feedback to the telephone care provider when a patient who was triaged over the phone is very ill, has an unusual or interesting problem, is admitted to the hospital, or could have been handled differently. In addition, if a telephone care provider consulted a physician about a particular call, the physician should provide feedback on the outcome of that call and what could be done differently, if anything. This helps the telephone care provider to recognize these patients in the future. If there are any untoward outcomes or outcomes for which there is an important lesson to be learned, the lesson should be shared as soon as possible with the telephone care provider involved, while the patient's presentation is fresh in her mind.

Develop an office environment that shares clinical material and provides feedback as a method of learning (being careful not to make the telephone care provider feel as though she is being criticized). It is very important to provide this type of feedback liberally, but diplomatically and kindly, during the telephone care provider's first 3 months on the job. If you plan to share the "case" with others during a telephone care meeting it is very important to do so anonymously.

Telephone Care Outcome File

Each case that is used as a teaching tool can be briefly summarized, along with the major teaching points, and placed in a telephone care outcome file. These educational telephone cases can be discussed at the next telephone care meeting in an anonymous fashion that will not make the telephone care providers feel like they are being put on the spot. These cases also can be used as "test cases" written up for the staff with the presenting symptoms and asking the staff to respond in writing. This information can be reviewed by the physician leader to determine if there is consistency among staff members in their responses to certain situations.

Telephone Care Outcome Log

For practices wanting to effectively manage a significant proportion of their patients over the phone without a visit, it may be worth the extra time and energy to keep a log of patients who receive triage and advice. Then the physician or mid-level practitioner who sees the patient in the office can put the diagnosis (or additional comments on whether the visit was necessary) on the log. The telephone care provider can review the log later to get a better sense of which patients really need to come in. The log becomes an easy means of providing feedback for the telephone care providers. A sample log is provided in Figure 14-1.

Follow-up Log

Another way to obtain feedback for telephone care providers is for them to place follow-up calls to check on the progress of the illness and the final outcome. The telephone care provider can call later in the day or the next day. The follow-up log (Figure 14-2) will remind her of the details of the problem at the time of the follow-up call. If the telephone care provider will not be at work at the time of the follow-up call, another telephone care provider can make the call and record details of the outcome for later review by the original telephone care provider.

Interesting or Difficult Call File

Telephone care providers often come across uncommon symptoms, unusual situations, difficult calls, or difficult callers. All of the telephone care providers will benefit from a discussion of how to handle these types of calls. These calls can be summarized and kept in a special call file. They can be discussed at a telephone care meeting, with all staff present. The discussion often will lead to new policies and procedures. It also is helpful to review calls together to discuss what symptom guideline to select on certain difficult calls.

Repeat Call File

There are some patients who are chronic frequent callers and some are frequent callers for a brief period around an acute issue. There should be a policy on acute frequent callers (eg, more than 2 calls in a 24-hour period). These patients should be seen because often the patient is more ill than appreciated over the phone or has a concern that has not surfaced yet. Chronic repeat callers often have underlying issues that have not been addressed. Their calls can be tracked and the caller can be discussed at the telephone care meeting, so that a plan can be formulated to better understand and manage the underlying issues.

Telephone Care Meetings

Telephone care meetings should be held in every practice and can be the forum in which QI activities and continuing education in telephone care occur. Telephone care meetings should be attended by the entire telephone care staff and the physician or mid-level practitioner who serves as medical director for telephone care. Although it often is helpful for a practice to designate a particular physician to this task, rotating this role among the physicians can be helpful in providing a variety of other perspectives.

The focus should be to create a positive learning environment and an open atmosphere in which everyone's contributions on how to improve services are appreciated. These meetings can include the following activities:

- Discuss lessons learned from an outcomes file.
- Discuss lessons learned from a complaint file.
- Discuss lessons learned from an interesting/difficult case file.
- Plan audits and discuss audit results.

- Discuss the telephone management of common clinical problems. This can be done by reviewing a guideline, emphasizing the knowledge behind the triage questions and dispositions.
- Discuss new developments in the literature or current controversies. These can be in the form of prepared talks or reviews of articles.
- Discuss possible new policies and standards or changes to old ones.

Telephone care meetings, and the QI process in general, will be most successful if the meetings are held on a regular basis. Monthly meetings enable prompt feedback and the ability to educate on recent trends of illnesses in the community. This interval is best suited for implementing new programs. As the telephone care program matures, telephone care meetings can be held every other month, or quarterly.

Figure 14-1. Sample Telephone Care Outcome Log

Patient Name	Date/Time of Call	Symptoms	Nurse Triage Disposition	Date/Time of Visit	Diagnosis	Comments

Figure 14-2. Sample Follow-up Log

Patient Name	Date/Time of Call	Symptoms	Reason for Follow-up	When to Follow-up	Date/Time of Follow-up	Outcome

Chapter 15

Managing the Demand for Visits Using Telephone Care

Although in many regions of the country managed care and capitation have not reached the levels that had been expected, there are many areas in which health plans provide inducements for practices to use the telephone to reduce use of expensive health care services, especially after hours. In addition, many family practices experience such high demand for office visits that they need to rigorously triage and advise over the phone to reduce office visit volumes. So, increasingly, the telephone is being used to manage the demand for office visits and emergency department (ED) visits by providing non-visit care.

There is certainly plenty of room for more vigorous telephone triage in most offices. There are several studies confirming that between 40% to 60% of scheduled visits during office hours could have been managed by phone. After hours, 50% to 60% of calls can be managed without a visit and another 20% to 30% can be deferred until the office is open. So, when a practice has demand for appointments that exceeds its capacity or more than 40% of patients in the practice are capitated, the practice will want to use rigorous triage and advice to manage patients over the phone during office hours. When a practice has more than 40% managed care contracts, after-hours calls should be rigorously triaged.

Rigorous Guidelines
The first step in providing rigorous telephone triage is to select telephone care guidelines that have been specifically designed to safely manage as many patients as is appropriate with home care instructions.

Two-Step Telephone Triage Process
The most efficient way to rigorously triage by telephone, yet minimize physician time on the phone, is to use a 2-step process. A physician can manage another 10% to 20% more patients without a visit than a nurse using telephone care guidelines. During office hours a physician can handle up to 60% to 70% and after hours up to 90% of clinical calls without a visit. When rigorous triage is needed, the physician should participate in the telephone care process. The nurse, using telephone care guidelines, provides the first step by handling all triage and advice calls. When the telephone guideline directs the telephone care provider to have the patient seen, rather than arranging a visit, she instead arranges for a physician to speak to the caller, thereby performing a second-level triage. This approach is particularly appropriate for after-hours telephone care that could result in an ED visit in practices with a high proportion of managed care patients. It is less practical for managing telephone care during office hours.

Three-Step Triage and Advice Process
Another approach to managing the demand for care is to reduce the number of phone calls by providing patients with materials they can use to answer common questions and even do self-triage. This step would become the first stage in a 3-stage process.

1. Self-triage and advice
2. Telephone nurse triage and advice
3. Physician triage and advice by telephone

Self-triage and advice can be provided in several different formats.

1. Practice handouts, given out at entry into the practice.
2. A book recommended for patients to purchase about illness or symptom management.
3. Practice Web site health information and triage and advice.

Patients will use these resources much more often if they are frequently reminded about them. The reception/scheduling staff and telephone care providers can respectfully ask if the caller has referred to these resources prior to calling. Also, it helps to have reminders in the examination room, in the practice newsletter, and on the recording that callers listen to while on hold.

Triage All Appointment Calls

This approach is the most aggressive of all of the options described in this chapter. When the need for rigorous telephone triage is very intense, some practices provide triage and advice to all callers requesting an appointment. However, if the caller still wants an appointment even after the telephone care provider has suggested self-care, it is a good policy to accommodate the request.

Risks of Using Telephone Triage to Manage Demand

There is a definite public backlash that has formed against limiting care by health plans or physicians. There has been recent legislation in most states requiring health plans and providers to allow patients to be seen if the caller perceives that he or she has an emergency. If a "prudent layperson" could consider the problem emergent, it is emergent. Therefore, telephone triage should be offered, not required. Malpractice juries have clearly shown their disapproval of attempts to use the telephone to limit care if there is a bad outcome. It is not wise to take chances. Nonphysician telephone care providers should not triage any more rigorously than the guidelines support. Patient safety always takes precedence. Caller comfort and satisfaction also should be strongly considered.

Chapter 16

Reimbursement for Telephone Care

Despite the fact that telephone care is increasing, requires a high level of skill, entails significant practice expenses, and carries high malpractice risks, telephone care has typically not been billed by physicians or reimbursed by health plans. This chapter provides an overview of the issues related to billing for telephone care and offers specific guidelines to physicians seeking reimbursement for telephone care.

Background

Until recently, little attention was focused on the issue of reimbursement for telephone care. As modern family practice evolved, physicians, patients, and payers seemed to accept the notion that in-office and after-hours telephone care was to be included at no extra charge as an adjunct to the medical services offered by physicians. This was possible in part because operating revenues from practices were often sufficient to cover the costs of telephone care.

During the development of Evaluation and Management (E/M) codes in the American Medical Association (AMA) *Current Procedural Terminology (CPT)* manual, some assumed that telephone care was bundled in the preservice and post-service times used in the Hsaio study to assign relative value units (RVUs) to *CPT* codes. Despite the fact that many of the assigned preservice and post-service times were not particularly representative of the telephone care provided by family physicians, telephone care was ultimately included in pre- and post-visit care. This argument has been used by many health plans to deny payments for these services, a decision that was reinforced when the Centers for Medicare and Medicaid Services (CMS) did not assign RVUs to case-management and care plan oversight services by telephone when these codes were developed and included in the *CPT* manual.

Over the past 5 years, a number of significant changes in family practice have prompted a reexamination of the issues related to reimbursement for telephone care. Busy families, many with both parents employed and increasingly using child care, have come to expect greater access to telephone advice. The advent of managed care and particularly a move to transfer the risks to the providers through capitation, put significant pressure on physicians to limit office and emergency department (ED) visits. This change emphasized the role of the telephone as a tool to limit use and health care costs. The increase in demand for telephone care has occurred at a time of declining reimbursement and increasing costs (immunizations, medications, documentation, and paperwork) in family physicians' offices. This combination has resulted in greater focus on the importance of reimbursement for telephone services. The need for increased documentation of all care provided, including telephone care, along with the time and expense required to meet these standards, has become increasingly burdensome. Finally, family physicians, while facing greater personal dissatisfaction in practice (in part related to the increasing burdens of telephone care, documentation, and paperwork), have turned to after-hours call centers in increasing numbers. The high cost and poor financial performance of these programs also have highlighted the need for a rational reexamination of the issues related to reimbursement for telephone care.

As all these trends have converged on family practice, physicians have been increasingly forced to consider reimbursement for telephone care in efforts to maintain profitability in their practices. Recent surveys have shown that developing RVUs to ensure adequate reimbursement for telephone care is supported by many family physicians. They argue that the physician work component of telephone care shares all the characteristics of in-office care, except for the hands-on physical examination. In support of this position, they point out that the CMS has already recognized the need to pay for services in which a physical examination is not performed (eg, telemedicine services) and developed a reimbursement formula for these services.

Although there seems to be support among physicians for seeking reimbursement for these important services, there are very limited data on the proportion of family practices that actually report and bill for these services. It is estimated that between 2% and 5% of family practices charge for telephone care. This low rate likely reflects frustration on the part of physicians, most of whom are aware of nonpayment (by payers) for telephone services and the fact that the actual cash collections for telephone care do not cover the billing and collection costs associated with submitting these claims.

Not all physicians, however, support billing patients and health plans for telephone services. Some have raised concerns that billing for telephone care may (1) deter poor families from calling with serious problems, (2) create a negative physician image, (3) tempt physicians to overuse (or abuse) the practice of charging for telephone care, and (4) possibly cause patients to switch their care to practices that do not charge for telephone care.

CPT Codes for Telephone Care

Case-Management Services
The AMA *CPT* manual, the standard reference for coding medical encounters with patients, categorizes telephone calls as either case-management or care plan oversight services. Telephone calls by physicians for case management (eg, management of an acute illness or injury, consultation with a family or another health care professional, coordination of care) are categorized by the complexity of medical decision making. Case-management telephone calls involving simple, intermediate, or complex decision making are described by *CPT* codes **99371, 99372,** and **99373,** respectively (Table 16-1). These codes can and should be used for initial patient evaluation or triage that requires clinical decision making. These codes also can be used for calls with other health professionals, including other physicians, nurses, physical therapists, or health care providers caring for the patient at home or in another care setting. For example, a brief call to a parent advising the parent of the results of a bilirubin test in a neonate after discharge from the nursery or a follow-up call to a family of an infant with diarrhea that results in advancement of formula would be coded using *CPT* code **99371.** An intermediate call providing triage and advice for home care of a child with a single day of diarrhea and vomiting would be coded using **99372.** A lengthy call with anxious or distraught parents who just discovered their adolescent to be using drugs may be coded using **99373.**

The issue of double payment (ie, the preservice component of an E/M code includes telephone care) does need resolution at a national level. Prior to resolving this dispute, one approach could be the following: If a patient call about a clinical problem is handled by a physician without a health care visit, it should be billed. If a patient's call leads to a visit, this

| | Table 16-1 | |
| | *CPT* Codes Used for Telephone Care—Case-Management Services | |
Code	Description	Examples
99371	Telephone call by physician to patient or health care professional for consultation, coordinating management—Simple or brief	Report a test result. Clarify/alter previous instructions. Integrate new information into plan. Adjust therapy.
99372	Telephone call by physician to patient or professional for consultation, management, or case coordination—Intermediate	Advice to established patient about new problem. Initiate therapy that can be handled by telephone. Coordinate management of new problem in established patient.
99373	Telephone call by physician to patient or professional for consultation, management, or case coordination—Complex or lengthy	Complex or lengthy counseling. Prolonged discussion with family. Lengthy communication necessary to coordinate complex care effort.

telephone call service would be included in the preservice component of the E/M code used for that office visit. When telephone discussion with other health professionals is required, these can be reported in addition to the office E/M code. For example, if a patient calls with a rash and the triage and advice provided results in a visit to the office, the call with the patient cannot be reported because it is part of pre-visit care. If, however, after seeing the patient the physician calls a dermatologist to discuss the rash and review the case and associated information, this call can be reported using *CPT* code **99371.** A call with a specialist concerning complex diagnoses, detailed review of laboratory results, or particularly complex management plans all would be reported using *CPT* codes **99372** or **99373.**

Care Plan Oversight Services
Telephone calls that are included within care plan oversight services reflect physician work in the complex and multidisciplinary management of patients cared for by a home health agency, hospice, or nursing facility. These calls can be reported using *CPT* codes **99374–99375** and **99377–99380** (Table 16-2), with *CPT* code **99374** used for calls of 15 to 29 minutes duration and **99375** for calls of 30 minutes or more. Only one physician may report services for a given period to reflect that physician's sole or predominant supervisory role with a particular patient. These codes should not be reported for supervision of patients under the care of home health agencies, unless they require consistent and repetitive supervision of therapy.

Care plan oversight services are cumulative over a 1-month period and categorized by physician time spent in providing telephone care. The inclusion of time spent as criteria for selecting a specific level of service for telephone care is unique and stands in contrast to other E/M codes, which are based on 2 or 3 (depending if it is a new or established visit)

	Table 16-2	
	CPT Codes Used for Telephone Care—Care Plan Oversight Services	
Code	**Description**	**Examples**
99374	Physician supervision of a patient under the care of a home health facility (patient not present) requiring coordination of multidisciplinary care. 15-29 minutes within a calendar month	Development or revision of care plans, review of reports or laboratory studies, communication (including phone calls) with other caregivers for assessment, care decisions, integrating new information, or adjustment of treatment plans or medical therapy.
99375	30 minutes or more within a calendar month	
99377	Physician supervision of a hospice patient (patient not present) requiring coordination of multidisciplinary care. 15-29 minutes within a calendar month	See **99374.**
99378	30 minutes or more within a calendar month	
99379	Physician supervision of a nursing facility patient (patient not present) requiring coordination of multidisciplinary care. 15-29 minutes within a calendar month	See **99374.**
99380	30 minutes or more within a calendar month	

essential elements, including history, physical examination, and medical decision making. Time is considered in selecting an E/M code only when counseling exceeds 50% of an E/M visit or prolonged physician attendance is required. For care plan oversight and case-management services, it should be noted that none of these telephone codes apply to telephone triage and advice provided by nurses.

Prolonged Services

If a telephone call lasts for more than 30 minutes, and if the physician sees the patient for a procedure or service the same day, physicians may report the call using the prolonged services *CPT* codes +**99358** and +**99359.** These codes are used to report the total duration of non–face-to-face time spent by a physician on a given date providing prolonged services. These add-on codes are only reported in addition to other physician services, including E/M services at any level. Use *CPT* code +**99358** to report the first hour of prolonged services on a given date or a total duration of prolonged service for 30 to 60 minutes on a given date. It may only be used once per date. Prolonged services of less than 30 minutes are not recorded. *CPT* code +**99359** can be reported for each subsequent 30 minutes of prolonged services after 75 minutes. Prolonged services less than 15 minutes beyond the first hour are not reported.

Telephone Calls and Hospital Care

The time spent during an encounter may not be used to determine the level of coding unless counseling, coordination of care, or both account for more than 50% of the face-to-face time with patients. Face-to-face time in outpatient visits is generally considered to be the amount of time the physician spends in the room with the patient. However, during hospital care, face-to-face time includes "floor" time spent by the physician on the inpatient unit, which can include time at the bedside as well as time spent writing notes, communicating with the family or other providers, and reviewing laboratory and diagnostic studies. In certain cases, especially in providing hospital care, if care coordination by telephone is required, a physician may wish to coordinate the patient's care (eg, speak with a consultant) while still on the inpatient unit and include the telephone care in the E/M service. In some cases, the extra time involved with the call, if it is documented and exceeds 50% of the face-to-face time, may allow the physician to report a higher level of service, assuming the history, examination, and medical decision making also justify the higher level of service. When compared to the uncertainty of receiving payment for the same call made later that day from the office and reported as a case-management service, this may be a favorable approach.

Documentation and Reporting

Reporting *CPT* codes for telephone care requires that the physician ensure appropriate documentation to support the level of service. However, unlike other E/M codes for which there are fairly specific guidelines for the various code descriptors, such as history, examination, and medical decision making, the *CPT* manual provides little specific guidance on the criteria to select between *CPT* codes **99371–99373.** For reporting all codes, we suggest that physicians include in their documentation template the following information, which may be used to justify their selection of a specific code:

- Type of patient.
  - New.
  - Established.
- Purpose of call.
  - Evaluate new problem and provide triage and/or advice.
  - Follow-up on a problem treated in the office, ED, or hospital.
  - Report results.
  - Coordinate management with other health professionals.
  - Clarify or adjust management plan for established problem.
- Complexity (based on the number of diagnoses or management options, amount of information reviewed, the risk of complication/morbidity, one versus several health professionals involved).
  - Minimal.
  - Low/moderate.
  - High.
- Total time spent providing telephone care (minutes).

As a reference, typical times for "established patient visit" E/M codes **99211, 99212,** and **99213** are 5, 10, and 15 minutes, respectively.

Fees for Telephone Care Services

Among physicians who support reimbursement for telephone services, there is a wide range of opinion about appropriate fees for telephone care. A survey of Albany, NY, physicians determined that most feel that physician calls should be reimbursed with a range of $2 to $2.50 per minute. A fee survey of 1,619 pediatricians conducted by the American Academy of Pediatrics (AAP) indicated physician charges of $20 for *CPT* telephone code **99371,** $30 for *CPT* code **99372,** and $50 for *CPT* code **99373.** In the absence of general consensus and established RVUs, deciding what to charge becomes a judgment call to be made by the physicians in the practice. A recent article published in *Pediatrics* recommended that physicians consider charging something in the range of $21 for **99371,** $32 for **99372,** and $52 for **99373.** For codes **99373–99376,** we recommend that physicians determine an hourly rate for telephone care and bill accordingly. Using an hourly telephone consultation rate of $100 per hour would result in a charge of $50 to $100 for code **99373,** depending on the time involved.

Billing and Collections for Telephone Care

Health Plans

Some Medicaid and other managed care plans include telephone triage as one of their covered services under capitation. Under these situations, physicians generally cannot bill for telephone services. For each capitated contract held, primary care physicians should confirm whether telephone calls are included in their capitation pool. In other situations, third-party payers also provide after-hours call services for patients, delivered through regional call centers and often without communication with the primary care physician. Physicians should be aware of these arrangements when negotiating contracts, as payers already providing telephone triage may be unwilling to reimburse primary care physicians for providing these same services. For patients covered under fee-for-service contracts, charges for telephone care should be submitted to payers using a CMS 1500 professional billing form. It is important to track reimbursement experience with each payer to determine the office experience with payments. This will raise awareness among payers and possibly help set the stage for reimbursement negotiations for this important component of patient care. Many plans (especially those serving Medicaid enrollees) will simply not pay for these services. Even in such cases a meticulous accounting of rejected telephone claims may be a valuable tool to raise awareness or as part of a reconciliation or contract negotiation process. For those that do pay, the collection rate from commercial insurers for telephone care charges has been reported in the range of 33% to 60%.

Patients

The topic of billing patients directly for telephone care is controversial. The AAP *Coding for Pediatrics 2001* manual recommends that to ensure that all patients being charged for telephone calls are treated equally and fairly, "the physician must be willing to (1) bill the patient for the service if the code is rejected by the insurance carrier and (2) charge a co-payment for the service."

There are few reports describing the perspective of families on payment for telephone care. One Colorado family physician group reports 28 years' experience charging for telephone care with very minimal patient complaints about the fee. Patient satisfaction with telephone triage and advice programs is generally very high. However, many patients also feel that they should not have to pay for this service. In a survey in Albany, NY, after-hours callers to a primary care practice indicated that they were willing to pay $25 per call to prevent a visit to an ED or perhaps to the office. If studies confirmed the efficacy and cost-effectiveness of these services, families might be less likely to object to paying for telephone care. Similarly, if the co-payments for office visits exceeded the costs of telephone care, patients may be more willing to pay cash for telephone services.

In certain circumstances, patients would rather spend time over the phone with their family physician than miss work for visits that may not require a physical examination, such as a behavioral program or asthma management. In some practices, physicians offer telephone case management as an alternative to office visits. Physicians who have used this approach successfully point out that the key is to clearly explain and define to the patients in advance of the telephone visit that the payer will not reimburse for this service and that the office will bill them directly for the telephone consultation.

Given the uncertainty and range of patient response to billing for telephone care, in all cases, physicians who choose to begin billing patients for telephone calls should be aware of a wide range of possible patient reaction and develop a communications plan and set expectations around billing for telephone care in a prospective fashion.

Services Provided by After-Hours Triage and Advice Centers

In many communities, physicians use the services of after-hours telephone triage and advice programs. These programs, often sponsored by hospitals, employ nurses who make use of computerized or written guidelines to triage calls from patients with medical complaints. Many (although not all) medical call centers charge physicians a monthly, or per-call, fee for triage services. Fees vary widely and are reported to range from $5 to $20 per call. There is little experience with directly billing the patients for services provided to them by after-hours call centers or passing the cost of triage services from the physician to patients. Physicians seeking to bill health plans for services provided by after-hours call centers are hampered by issues of documentation and the fact that these services often are provided by nurses, while the *CPT* codes for telephone care do not include nurse triage and advice. There are anecdotal reports of physicians billing patients directly for services provided by after-hours call centers, including some who claim to have high collection rates for these services. Before embarking on this approach, physicians should carefully review health plan contracts to ensure there are no prohibitions against direct billing for telephone services provided by them or after-hours call programs.

Alternatives to Charging for Telephone Care

Some physicians may choose not to charge health plans or patients directly for telephone care and instead seek additional capitation payments or increased office charges to offset the costs of telephone care. Because few payers presently adjust payments based on charges, increasing charges may not be particularly effective in increasing revenue. Based on managed care and fee-for-service practice survey data, the total office costs of telephone care for a typical family practice are approximately $3 per visit and typical capitation-based telephone costs are approximately $1 per member per month.

CPT 5-digit codes, nomenclature, and other data are copyright 2002 American Medical Association. All Rights Reserved. No fees, schedules, basic units, relative values, or related listings are included in *CPT*. The AMA assumes no liability for the data contained herein.

Chapter 17

Staffing and Retention of Good Staff

Determining Staffing Needs

Payroll expense for telephone care providers and reception/scheduling staff typically accounts for more than 90% of the budget for telephone care. To be cost-efficient, staffing decisions should be based on the telephone care objectives, call volumes, and call duration (or calls per hour) for your particular practice. It is important to remember that call volumes and staffing objectives vary greatly from practice to practice. To assist your efforts an example of how to determine staffing needs is provided later in this chapter.

Telephone Care Objectives

Objectives will vary from practice to practice and within a practice depending on time of year. What are your primary objectives for telephone care? Do you want to provide telephone triage and advice only for those callers who specifically request it, or do you want to provide telephone triage and advice for all calls about acute illness to reduce the number of office visits (as in a practice that is 40% capitated or more, or a practice in an underserved area that sees too many patients each day)? Do you need to fill your office appointment schedule or thin it out? Do you want to respond immediately to all clinical calls or are you willing to have some or all of the callers who want telephone care wait for a callback? Do you need to focus on improving callback times to improve caller satisfaction? What level of personnel is available in your community and what is the usual pay range? How much are you willing to pay to meet these objectives? Answering these questions is the first step in determining staffing for telephone care.

Direct Calls Versus Callbacks

If your staffing objectives include allowing callbacks for telephone care, you can staff at a lower level, perhaps 66% to 75% of the staff compared to the number of staff needed to handle all calls directly the moment they come in. For example, assume that in your office a telephone care provider can handle 8 triage and advice calls per hour. And assume that the call volume data you collected on telephone triage and advice calls show that normally there are 13 telephone care calls between 8:00 and 9:00 am, 6 calls between 9:00 and 10:00 am, 4 calls between 10:00 and 11:00 am, and 8 calls between 11:00 am and 12:00 noon for a total of 31 calls in 4 hours. This volume can be managed by one telephone care provider, allowing for callbacks. Not everyone who calls in the first hour will be handled in the first hour; but, if you take messages, everyone will receive a callback within an hour or so. If you want to answer all calls as they come in, you need 2 telephone care providers the first hour, and the telephone care provider for 2 of the next 3 hours will be underused.

We recommend staffing at a level such that you will have enough telephone care providers for most hours, and that you anticipate that there will not be quite enough during the high-volume hours, but they will be able to catch up during subsequent hours. The most time-efficient approach to taking messages for the telephone care provider is to use voice mail, to which the receptionist can transfer the call. The recorded prompt on the telephone voice mail can provide directions about what information to leave for the telephone care provider, an anticipated length of time until callback, and an invitation to press zero to get back to the receptionist if the caller feels the problem is more urgent.

Call Volume Data

Collecting data on the calls to your practice for telephone care is time-consuming and may not seem cost-efficient. However, the information derived from determining call volumes can prove vital to your efforts to determine the most efficient approach to staffing. The telephone care providers have an intuitive sense of the call volumes. They know that the peak hours are first thing in the morning and first thing in the afternoon, with other smaller peaks just before lunch and late afternoon. They know Mondays seem to be the busiest day. But if you want to contain costs, you need to know your telephone care demand by hour of day, day of week, and season. If you collect these data regularly (during 1 week in each quarter), you can adapt your staffing to the changes in volumes and reduce costs while maintaining caller satisfaction.

Call Duration and Calls Per Hour

Call duration and calls per hour are important measures of efficiency. Chapter 6 emphasizes the importance of defining the components of a model call and working to make each component of the call time-efficient. Reducing the call duration (while maintaining quality of care and caller satisfaction) is the key personnel management challenge. The next most important challenge is to staff so that you have enough telephone care providers to handle the volume of calls. With your best telephone care providers, define a model call and observe how long it takes for them on average to complete each element of the call. You can use this information to establish a target clinical call duration (an ideal time and acceptable range). Performance evaluations, raises, and bonuses can depend to some degree on meeting acceptable average call duration. Acceptable call duration also can be used to make staffing decisions. If you determine that the average telephone triage and advice call in your practice takes 6 minutes, then you will expect the telephone care provider to handle 9 calls an hour. Remember, too, that 25% to 33% of the calls may be for health information only, which usually take only 3 to 4 minutes each. Perhaps (given the specific demands of your practice) the telephone care provider can handle 10 to 11 calls per hour (2-3 health information calls = 8-12 minutes and 8 triage calls = 48 minutes). And, of course, you need to factor in time for breaks. It is safe to assume a volume of 8 to 10 calls per hour.

Using the anticipated call volumes per hour and expected abilities of the telephone care staff to handle a certain number of calls per hour, you can determine how many telephone care providers you are likely to need hour by hour. Because the number of telephone care providers needed will likely vary each hour, you can plan for the telephone care provider to perform other functions during the anticipated downtimes.

Example of Collecting and Using Call Data to Plan Staffing

There are wide variations in the number of telephone calls to family practices, depending on the age distribution of the patient population, practice philosophy of the physician, socioeconomic status of the patients, and whether the practice is urban or rural. So, there is no "average" call volume for a family practice. The following is an example of how a family practice can collect and use data to plan staffing: A 4-physician, urban family practice currently does not have an organized telephone triage and advice system in place. Triage and advice is done mostly by licensed practical nurses (LPNs) and medical assistants (MAs). The practice has a head nurse who is a registered nurse and supervises the LPNs and MAs. Whoever is available to take calls, including reception staff, gives health information and, at times, even does telephone triage. The physicians have asked the head nurse to develop a telephone triage and advice system. They want it to be cost-effective. This particular practice is in an underserved area and has a very high volume of visits. Patients are encouraged to call for triage and advice before scheduling a visit.

It is estimated that the practice gets around 60,000 calls to the practice each year, of which approximately 12,000 are of a clinical nature (roughly 8,000 for telephone triage and advice and 4,000 for health information only). Of the clinical calls, about 8,000 occur during office hours and 4,000 occur after hours. These estimates are extrapolated from data collected during an average week in the spring. Table 17-1 shows call volume data collected during that week by day of week and hour of day.

The physicians use this information to plan for front desk reception and schedule staffing. They next determine which of the calls involved clinical care by telephone (Table 17-2).

Table 17-1 Data on All Calls to a 4-Physician Denver, CO, Family Practice During a Week in March						
Hours	**Monday**	**Tuesday**	**Wednesday**	**Thursday**	**Friday**	**Saturday**
8:00–9:00 am	59	32	40	36	39	12
9:00–10:00 am	51	41	33	37	37	10
10:00–11:00 am	45	32	26	29	27	8
11:00 am–12:00 noon	41	34	27	31	26	7
12:00 noon–1:00 pm	15	9	8	11	8	6
1:00–2:00 pm	31	33	34	14	28	0
2:00–3:00 pm	37	25	19	25	27	0
3:00–4:00 pm	29	29	20	22	22	0
4:00–5:00 pm	26	26	23	19	23	0
5:00–6:00 pm	8	8	4	4	6	0
Total	342	269	234	228	243	43

Table 17-2 Data on All Clinical Calls to a 4-Physician Denver, CO, Family Practice During a Week in March						
Hours	**Monday**	**Tuesday**	**Wednesday**	**Thursday**	**Friday**	**Saturday**
8:00–9:00 am	10	5	7	5	6	3
9:00–10:00 am	9	6	5	6	5	2
10:00–11:00 am	8	5	4	5	5	2
11:00 am–12:00 noon	6	5	4	4	4	1
12:00 noon–1:00 pm	2	2	2	2	2	2
1:00–2:00 pm	5	7	6	4	4	0
2:00–3:00 pm	6	4	5	5	4	0
3:00–4:00 pm	4	4	4	4	5	0
4:00–5:00 pm	4	4	3	4	4	0
5:00–6:00 pm	2	2	1	1	2	0
Total	56	44	41	40	41	10

Using the numbers in Table 17-2, they calculate how many telephone care providers they would need each hour during an average week in the spring, assuming that each provider could handle 8 calls per hour (Table 17-3). This was done by dividing the average number of calls each hour of the week by 8.

Because the physicians in the practice are willing to have callbacks for triage and advice calls, they decide to staff Monday mornings with one telephone care nurse, recognizing that she may not be able to handle all calls in the first few hours but will catch up as the morning progresses. For Tuesday through Friday, there will be times when a full nurse will be needed; for other hours, a nurse can work in other office duties with clinical calls. Saturday mornings each of the nurses involved in office visits pitch in with calls for telephone care.

Adapting to the Seasons
Most practices find that call volumes in the slowest weeks in the summer are 65% to 70% of the volumes in the busiest weeks in the winter. So they adapt their staffing to the season. In the case of the 4-physician family practice in this example, one telephone care provider may be needed all day during January and February. During the summer, the nurse assigned to clinical telephone calls may be able to perform other duties during all hours. In fact, some of the nursing staff may be able to take off June, July, and August.

Table 17-3 **Calculation of Number of Telephone Care Nurses to Handle Clinical Calls** **by Hour of Day and Day of Week in March**						
Hours	**Monday**	**Tuesday**	**Wednesday**	**Thursday**	**Friday**	**Saturday**
8:00–9:00 am	1.25	0.5	1	0.5	2	0.5
9:00–10:00 am	1.25	1	0.5	1	1	0.25
10:00–11:00 am	1	0.5	0.5	0.5	1	0.25
11:00 am–12:00 noon	0.25	0.5	0.5	0.5	1	0.125
12:00 noon–1:00 pm	1	0.25	0.25	0.5	0.5	0.25
1:00–2:00 pm	1	1	0.5	0.5	1	0
2:00–3:00 pm	1	0.5	0.5	1	1	0
3:00–4:00 pm	0.5	0.5	0.5	1	1	0
4:00–5:00 pm	0.25	0.25	0.25	1	1	0
5:00–6:00 pm	0.5	0.5	0.25	0.125	0.125	0

Other Staffing Tips

Telephone care can be stressful during high-volume times and always requires a high degree of concentration. Experienced telephone care providers in larger practices say it is difficult to maintain that level of concentration all day. The ideal shift duration appears to be 4 hours. If a telephone care provider will be covering an entire day at 8 calls per hour, it is important to build in 5 minutes per hour away from the phones and a 1-hour break away from phones in the middle of the day.

A very common method for staffing low-volume hours is to have the office nurse do call-backs between her other patient-related duties. Most family practices with 8 or fewer physicians can assign other tasks to the nurse who handles clinical calls. As the hourly volumes increase to a point at which this is not possible, the telephone care provider's primary role would be telephone care. Other duties can be worked in to hours with low call volume, such as referrals, filling in for other staff during breaks, follow-up calls, and reminder calls.

Another strategy for small practices is to promote the concept of telephone care hours, limiting telephone triage and advice or health information calls to specific hours, perhaps 8:00 to 10:00 am, 1:00 to 2:00 pm, and 3:30 to 4:30 pm. This information would be included in the practice telephone policy, handbook, and information message that callers listen to on the automated telephone attendant or while on hold. Callers requesting telephone care would be asked if they could wait until those hours for a return call. If the caller indicates that the problem requires a more urgent response, he or she would be accommodated.

Another option to keep in mind is remote telephone care staffing. For telephone care during office hours, it is appropriate for only special situations because it is relatively inefficient. You might consider having a telephone care provider take clinical calls from home if, for example, she has a condition requiring bed rest or if a family member is at home requiring supervision. In this situation, a special accommodation can be made so that remote telephone care is possible. When telephone care providers are taking calls after hours, taking remote calls from home is ideal. (See Chapter 21.)

Retention of Telephone Care Staff

A skilled telephone care provider is a treasure for a practice. It is a very important service to the patients. Training of the telephone care provider is an enormous investment of time and resources for the practice, so it is very important to retain the skilled telephone care provider. There are many factors involved in encouraging skilled providers to remain with a practice.

Create a Flexible, Desirable Job
- Telephone care is a good role for a nurse with a disability, those approaching retirement, working parents who want to work part-time, or people who want to work 9 months per year.
- Meet with the telephone care providers in your practice, listen to their opinions on how to retain good providers, and seriously consider their suggestions.
- Telephone care lends itself to working 4-hour shifts. Be flexible by scheduling to meet special needs.
- Office nurses often prefer the variety of a job that combines telephone care and patient care.

Show How Much the Position and Person Are Valued
- Develop a separate, specific identity for the staff who do telephone care, as though it is a specialty with special status.
- Regularly verbally acknowledge the high level of skill required for the position and provide a higher salary for staff who do telephone care.
- When providing feedback, focus on what can be learned rather than criticizing.
- Be sure at least one of the physicians show his or her appreciation for this position in the office by always attending the telephone care quality improvement (QI) and continuing education meeting.
- Periodically write a thank-you note to each telephone care provider.

Enable Providers to Maintain Their Professional Skills
- Support, enable, and fund attendance at telephone care QI meetings.
- Assign administrative tasks in telephone care to telephone care providers (eg, audits).
- Offer opportunities to attend telephone care workshops.
- Develop an environment in which sharing cases for learning purposes is encouraged and people do not feel criticized.

Improve the Comfort and Reduce the Stress of the Position

- Create a pleasant, quiet, calm working environment for the telephone care providers, with enough privacy to allow for confidential conversations.
- Be willing to provide an ergonomically appropriate chair, desk, footrest, phone, and headset.
- Allow the option for telephone care providers to take on different roles in the practice to maintain clinical skills and allow for a variety of activities.
- Ensure physician backup is readily available, pleasant, and supportive.
- HAVE FUN ON THE JOB!

Chapter 18

Understanding Telephone-Related Expenses in a Family Practice

The number of telephone calls to family practices varies greatly from practice to practice, depending on whether the physicians provide obstetric and pediatric care and on the proportion of geriatric patients and patients with chronic diseases. The annual call volume can range from 12,000 to 20,000 calls per physician in the practice. The average family practice in Colorado handles roughly 15,000 telephone calls per year per physician at a cost of approximately $18,000 per physician per year. The number of calls during which clinical care is provided appears to be increasing compared to studies in family practice in the 1970s and 1980s. On average, clinical calls account for 15% to 18% of all calls, yet they account for 30% of all telephone expenses. When the expenses of after-hours telephone care are added to office-hours telephone clinical care, the percentage of telephone expenses that are related to clinical care by telephone increases to more than 60%. Unfortunately, these telephone clinical contacts are not reimbursed, so a cost-efficient system for managing clinical care by telephone is imperative. And because medicolegal risk is increasing, it is important to balance expense, quality of care, and caller satisfaction. This chapter describes telephone expenses in a typical family practice. Chapter 19 presents strategies for managing clinical and nonclinical calls in a cost-efficient manner.

The first step in planning a more cost-efficient telephone care system is to understand the volume, flow, content, and expenses associated with calls managed by office staff. Because there are wide variations in these parameters among practices, your cost-efficiency planning will be most effective if you collect data in your own practice. Usually, your telephone service provider can provide you with data on call volume and flow (eg, number of calls, calls per hour, call duration, number of rings before a call is answered, call abandonment rate). If you have an automated attendant, voice mail, or a fax machine, you can obtain additional data on call flow from these sources. Simple office audits can determine whether the frequency of various reasons for calls resemble those described in the literature. Expenses can be calculated by a practice businessperson using personnel salaries, call volumes, call durations, and known fixed telephone expenses.

This chapter presents a summary of the medical and practice management literature and a study of telephone-related expenses conducted in selected Colorado family practices.

Call Volume
Call volume from the Colorado family practice study is summarized in Table 18-1. Call volume by hour of the day can be estimated using Table 17-1 in Chapter 17. The number of clinical calls can be estimated using data in Table 17-2 in Chapter 17.

Call Duration
The average call duration is 3 minutes for all calls during office hours. Telephone calls take more than 14 hours a week of staff time per physician in the practice, or 720 hours a year

Table 18-1 Typical Call Volumes From a Typical Colorado Family Practice (Actual Data From Your Practice May Vary.)		
Telephone Contacts per Physician in the Practice	**Per Week**	**Per Year***
During office hours	283	14,700
Administrative calls	235	12,200
Clinical calls	48	2,500
After hours	14	700
Clinical calls	12-13	650
Administrative calls	1-2	50
Total calls	297	15,000

*Approximation.

per physician in the practice. Table 18-2 shows the call duration for different types of office staff during office hours.

Telephone Expenses

The cost of personnel time in handling phone calls (including amortized capital costs and other monthly telephone expenses) accounts for 70% of all telephone-related expenses. Table 18-2 shows the average cost per call handled by each type of personnel. Time required to put documentation in the medical record is not included.

Table 18-3 summarizes telephone-related expenses, categorized as capital expenses, personnel expenses, and all other expenses. They are expressed as yearly expenses and expenses per call. Capital costs are one-time purchases of relatively expensive equipment. New, modern equipment can cost as much as $5,000 per physician in the practice. For low-end, used equipment, the cost can be held down to $500 per physician. The monthly, non-personnel costs include monthly telephone bill, paging service, cellular phone costs, answering service, fax machine, and malpractice costs (with the help of a malpractice carrier, we estimated the portion of the malpractice premium allocated to telephone care).

If the total telephone-related expense for services during office hours is annualized, the average cost for telephone services provided during office hours would be expected to be about $18,000 per physician in the practice per year, approximately $60 for each day the practice is open. After-hours telephone services add additional costs that are difficult to estimate because most physicians have trouble quantifying the value of their after-hours time and energy.

Table 18-2 Duration of Calls and Expense of Staff Time Spent Providing Telephone Service, by Type of Practice Staff Member				
Office Personnel	**Average Length of Call (Minutes)**	**% Office Hours Calls Handled**	**Average Cost/Call All Phone Expenses***	**% of Telephone Personnel Costs**
Receptionist/scheduler	2.6	57	$0.81	29
Business office, referral coordinator, insurance	3.6	16	$1.15	12
Nursing Staff (eg, licensed practical nurses, registered nurses, medical assistants	4.0	18	$1.26	14
Mid-level practitioners	3.8	2	$2.33	3
Physicians	3.9	7	$10.71	42
Total (average)	3		$1.25	

*Includes amortized capital costs, malpractice, and other monthly telephone expenses.

Table 18-3 All Telephone Expenses for Office Hours Only		
Average Expense Per Physician in Practice	**Per Year**	**Per Call**
Capital expenses (amortized over 5 years)	$800*	$0.06
Expense of personnel time on the phone	$12,600	$0.80
Other expenses of telephone-related services (eg, phone bill, answering service, cellular phones, pagers, portion of malpractice premiums)	$4,600	$0.38
Total	$18,000/y $1,500/mo $60/d	$1.24

*Range: $300–$1,000.

The Expense of Providing Clinical Care by Telephone

In the average family practice, telephone clinical care is defined as a telephone call that provides clinical triage, advice, health information, or teaching. Telephone clinical care is provided during 15% to 18% of office-hours calls; of these, two thirds provide triage and advice and one third provide teaching or health information. When a practice needs to actively reduce the number of appointments (either because its patient population is capitated or because it has too high a demand for visits to be handled by its resources), a family practice may handle twice that many clinical calls per year per physician. During office hours, there is a wide variation among practices in who handles clinical calls. Virtually all types of staff members get involved in triage and advice or health education in one practice or another, including reception staff and the business manager in some practices.

Another 29% of calls are related to clinical issues but do not involve clinical care per se: calling in prescriptions (20%), providing test results (4%), ordering tests (2%), arranging for medical equipment or home care (2%), and making arrangements with nursing homes (1%). Approximately 60% of clinical calls lead to an appointment, although only 30% to 40% actually need an appointment, according to the primary care physicians who were asked to assess the need.

The average and median call duration for all clinical calls are 5 minutes, with a range of 2 to 20 minutes. The average call for health information is 3 to 4 minutes; the average call for telephone triage and advice is 5 to 8 minutes. The average time in the practice devoted to telephone clinical care during office hours is 4 hours a week per physician in the practice. Add to this an additional 1 to 2 hours of after-hours telephone clinical care per physician per week in the practice; the total is 5 to 6 hours of clinical care provided by the practice per family physician per week, or between 250 and 300 hours per year.

Table 18-4 shows the cost per call for each type of office staff member. The total cost for clinical telephone care during office hours for a year is estimated to be $6,750 per physician in the practice per year. Another $5,270 will be spent on calls related to clinical issues (eg, prescriptions, test results, ordering tests, arranging medical equipment, home care, nursing homes). The cost of the average clinical call during office hours, $2.70, may seem lower than expected; this is because non-registered nurses provide much of the clinical care. In addition to these costs, there are approximately 700 additional clinical calls per year (between 55 and 60 hours) per physician in the practice managed after hours.

Call Distribution and Flow

Table 18-2 shows the percentage of all phone calls that various staff members handle and the relative expense. Although the front desk staff handles more than half of the calls, they represent less than 30% of the telephone staff costs. Physicians, on the other hand, handle only 7% of the calls but account for 42% of the personnel costs associated with the telephone.

Sixty-two percent of calls are incoming. The average call duration for incoming calls is 2.5 minutes and for outgoing calls is 3.5 minutes. Table 18-5 shows the reasons for calls. Fifty-four percent of calls are nonclinical and 46% have some clinical association (16% actual care by telephone). Nearly one fourth of all calls are related to making appointments: 15% making appointments (mostly incoming), 6% confirming appointments (nearly all of which are

Table 18-4 Expense Associated With Clinical Calls		
Staff Member	**Cost per Clinical Call**	**Average Clinical Call Duration (Minutes)**
Physician	$12.50	5.7
Mid-level practitioner	$2.90	5.8
Registered nurse	$1.75	5
Licensed practical nurse	$1.50	5
Medical assistant	$1.25	4.5
Estimated total (based on current distribution)	$2.70	5

outgoing), 2% canceling appointments, and 1% rescheduling. Nearly 10% of incoming calls are for nonmedical information.

Thirteen percent of calls are either transferred (8%) or a message is taken (5%). Table 18-6 shows the distribution of the transfer or message calls. Of these transfer or message calls, 90% are incoming calls handled by the receptionist and therefore potentially could be handled by an automated attendant and voice messaging system. Of those calls that potentially could be handled with an automated system, the cost in personnel time is $2,400 per physician in the practice per year.

Prescription refills account for 16% of calls. New prescriptions represent 4% of calls and mostly are handled by nurses and physicians. The cost to handle prescription refills is estimated at $3,000 per family physician in the practice per year. Results of laboratory and x-ray tests are given during 4% of calls.

On 3% of all calls, a staff member is placed on hold, for an average length of time of 4 minutes, amounting to 2 hours per month (24 hours per year) per physician in the practice. When annualized, the estimated cost associated with waiting on hold amounts to more than $400 per year per physician in the practice. Seventy-two percent of the time and expense is due to being on hold with health plans (average time of 5.7 minutes and range of 2-23 minutes), with 12% due to other health professionals (mostly pharmacists) and 14% for patients. One percent of calls receives a busy signal and 1% no answer.

Table 18-5 Reasons for Calls	
Reason for Call	**% of All Calls**
Appointment	24
Nonmedical information	9
Transfer call to someone in office	8
Message taken	5
Clinical call (health education or triage and advice)	16
Phone consultation obtained	1
New prescription	4
Prescription refill	16
Test result	4
Order/schedule test	2
Medical equipment, home care, nursing home	3
Business	2
Insurance, authorization, referral	5
Personal	1

Table 18-6 Call Transfers and Messages Taken for Types of Practice Staff Members		
Personnel	**% of All Transferred Calls to This Person**	**% of Messages Taken for This Person**
Telephone nurse (eg, licensed practical nurse, registered nurse, medical assistant)	29	36
Physician	20	33
Business office, manager	10	6
Referral staff	7	5
Mid-level practitioner	5	3
Medical records	2	3
Reception/scheduling	20	11
Personal/other	7	3

Chapter 19

Developing a Cost-effective Telephone Care System in the Office

A review of the data on telephone-related expenses presented in Chapter 18 suggests a variety of strategies for reducing the cost of telephone care and telephone-related activities in general. This chapter describes strategies in telephone care first, then strategies for reducing the cost of other telephone-related activities.

Strategies for Reducing the Expense of Clinical Care by Telephone

Delegating Calls

Delegating triage and advice calls and health information calls during office hours reduces expenses and improves call flow, office patient flow, and provider satisfaction. Routine clinical calls should be delegated to someone other than physicians or mid-level practitioners. Physicians and mid-level practitioners should handle only the more complicated clinical calls. Deciding which level of nurse to hire will depend on the finances and philosophy within the practice. Table 18-4 in Chapter 18 can help in the financial portion of the decision. It shows how much an average clinical call costs for each different type of office staff. At the present time, delegating routine telephone triage and advice to the most clinically experienced person the practice can afford is recommended.

Physician Calls

Physician calls should be limited to those clinical calls for which the nurse is concerned or uncertain, the nurse is directed by the telephone guideline, there is an apparent emergency, the call is from the hospital, the history is complicated, the patient or caller insists on speaking to the physician, the patient has a complicated problem or chronic disease, the call is coming late in the day and a visit would have to be arranged after hours, or the call is from another health care professional. Office staff should be provided with a list of the types of calls that should be transferred to a physician. Calls that can be handled by a nonphysician include referrals to other offices when not specifically speaking to the doctor at that office, laboratory reports, x-ray reports, durable medical equipment, use of home health care services, authorization for managed care of specific referrals and hospitalizations, prescription refills, and general health maintenance questions. Calls that can be deferred include patient inquiries, patient follow-ups, personal calls, and business calls. If calls from family members are transferred, they should be answered promptly by the physician. (A physician who repeatedly ignores general pages that a loved one is on hold does not promote a positive image.) The calls that are deferred can be batched for callback when possible and overseen by an experienced nurse who can prioritize them. Batched calls can be returned during specific 15-minute blocks built into the appointment schedule, 1 mid-morning and 1 mid-afternoon. Patient charts should be available for all physician calls because those will be the highest risk. If physician calls are not returned immediately, the caller should be given some expectation about the timing of a return call based on usual practice parameters. The office staff should record the time at which the patient or caller will be available for the physician's return call.

Call Length

Shortening the length of clinical calls is an important cost-saving measure. Establish a suggested target call duration and a target for the number of calls per hour, which can be built into standards of performance. (See Chapter 7.) Give appointments on demand and do not try to triage a call if the patient wants an appointment. When using telephone care guidelines, the nurse should stop asking questions when she gets to the first positive response that tells her what disposition to recommend. Do not ask any further questions if additional questions will not change the disposition of the call. It also is helpful to have a policy to avoid counseling patients on behavioral problems for more than 5 minutes. Anything more than that should be handled with an appointment. Document calls on log sheets that incorporate checklists and require little writing. (See Chapter 4.) When documenting the advice given, simply indicate which guideline was used and write or check a box indicating "per guideline." Consider providing (and referring patients to) handout materials. Illness handouts also can be made available on practice Web sites.

Reducing the Number of Clinical Calls

Reducing the number of clinical calls also can be accomplished using handouts, practice booklets, videotapes, audiotapes, prerecorded telephone messages, Web-based health information, and Web-based triage and advice for patients. Sixty percent of clinical calls to a family practice could be managed by the patient without a telephone call if health education materials are made available to patients.

Patient Education Handouts

The success of using handouts to reduce telephone calls has been described in the medical literature. The most cost-efficient approach is for the practice to recommend a book for families to purchase that covers common illnesses. Another method is to purchase a book of patient handouts and photocopy the ones on common problems to distribute to patients at health maintenance visits. The most cost-effective handout to give to all patients is one with dosages of all of the commonly used over-the-counter medications.

Health Information Messages

Prerecorded, audiotaped health information messages can be made available on automated systems to be accessed by patients using a touch-tone telephone. The patient receives from his or her primary care physician a printed directory with the phone number for the health information line and the specific touch-tone code numbers of the desired topics. The primary advantage of this technology is that it is caller-controlled, which makes it available at the moment of need, readily accessible, convenient, and confidential. Studies have shown that when all members of the practice actively encourage this approach, 60% of patients who use the system report that it prevented a call to the office. When this type of system is made available to your practice by a local hospital or other resource at no cost to your practice, it makes sense to use it. The expense of the hardware and licensing of the software make it difficult for any but the very largest practices to afford to buy it on their own. If a local hospital charges you for this service, it probably is not worth the expense unless you will aggressively encourage patients to use it.

Practice Web Sites

Practice Web sites are becoming popular and are usually provided by Internet companies or hospitals at no charge to practices. A recent study conducted in Colorado using Web-based triage and advice for patients has shown that 60% of patients who used the Web-based triage and advice were able to avoid calling the office.

The key to getting patients to use any of these patient education methods is to actively promote them. This can be accomplished by having reception staff and nurses remind patients about the availability of handouts, prerecorded messages, or the information on the Web site and by regularly referring patients to them as a source of triage and advice.

Cross-Training

Cross-training is another important strategy for reducing expenses. Many practices employ a variety of types of personnel including mid-level practitioners, registered nurses, licensed practical nurses, medical assistants, and health assistants. Each type of office staff member will be underused at times. It is cost-efficient to train and prepare each level of personnel to do telephone care so that they can assist the regular telephone care staff in managing the telephone care demand. However, it is equally important to be sure that they perform telephone care duties often enough (at least 16 hours per month) to maintain their skills.

Streamline Appointment Scheduling

Another cost-reduction strategy is to streamline appointment scheduling so the telephone care provider does not lose precious time away from telephone care. It is ideal for the telephone care provider to have immediate access to an automated scheduling system with same-day appointment slots available. If scheduling is done manually with a simple appointment book, callers who need appointments should be transferred to the scheduler. It is ideal in larger practices to have the schedulers and telephone care providers working in proximity to each other, away from the front desk.

Compensation

Telephone care provider compensation varies dramatically by region and in proportion to professional training. It is important to reward telephone care skill to retain good telephone care providers. One strategy for cost containment is to compensate telephone care providers on a per-call basis. This method is very appropriate for telephone care providers who take calls after hours. (See Chapter 22.) It is appropriate for those special instances when the telephone care provider handles calls from home during office hours. The method for calculating compensation on a per-call basis is described in Chapter 22.

Telephone Policies for Patients

An important step in improving cost-efficiency in telephone care is to educate patients about the services provided by telephone and how best to use them. Providing patients with a copy of the practice telephone policies will improve caller satisfaction, patient cooperation with your telephone cost-containment efforts, and time-efficiency for office staff. A sample 1-page handout is shown in Chapter 13. The practice telephone policy can be made available as a handout for all patients, as a prerecorded automated information line message, and on the practice Web site. It can include information on how to use the telephone for emergencies, after-hours calls, prescription refills, preferred times to call for advice and triage, obtaining information, or handling business or referral issues. It also can describe what information to have available during calls for advice. Caller ID with a blocking function is becoming an increasing problem for physicians returning calls to patients. To minimize this problem, instruct your staff to post signs in the office telling the patients to unblock their phones when expecting a return call. You also can include this request in your telephone policy statement.

Strategies for Reducing the Expense of Nonclinical Calls

Managing nonclinical call flow is an important cost-management strategy. The most common reasons for nonclinical calls are shown in Table 18-5 in Chapter 18. Table 18-6 in Chapter 18 shows the percentages of calls for each practice member for whom messages were taken or the call was transferred.

Strategies should be sought to reduce the number, duration, and expense of these common types of calls. Reception/scheduling staff should be given scripts for common types of calls and trained to make the appointment call as efficient as possible. Automated telephone systems, such as an automated attendant, voice mail, faxing, prerecorded lines, automated outbound call systems, and e-mail, can improve cost-efficiency.

Automated Telephone Systems

Automated attendant is an automated telephone call transferring and messaging system. Callers can select an automated transfer to a person, a prerecorded message, or an extension at which to leave a voice message. Because 13% of calls in a family practice either are transferred or have a message taken, automation of these 2 functions holds considerable promise for improving cost-efficiency. An automated attendant and voice messaging system has the potential to reduce the total number of calls handled by a person by 15%, which could reduce expenses by $2,800 per year per physician in the practice. The cost of an automated attendant/voice messaging system in Colorado is approximately $350 per year.

Tables 18-5 and 18-6 in Chapter 18 can be used to guide decisions about the organization of the automated attendant. Current business standards for automated attendant and voice mail systems should include the following features:

- The option to speak to a person (especially in clinical settings)
- Advice for callers about what to do in an emergency
- Last no longer than 20 seconds
- Have no more than 6 choices for callers to select from the main menu
- Involve no more than 2 levels of choices
- Must allow the provider to quickly recognize a malfunction in the system

A common order for listing options on an automated attendant in a family practice office (after the emergency disclaimer) is

1. Another health care professional calling
2. Triage and advice for acute illness
3. Appointment
4. Prescription refill
5. Test results
6. Business office and practice information

Automated messages should provide an indication of when to expect a return call. Menus should always have an opt-out feature for the impatient caller ("If you wish to speak to a staff person, press 0"). Directions should be short and simple to avoid confusing and frustrating the caller. Emergency instructions should be first on the menu. Try to avoid menu choices that prompt patients to dial other numbers, except in the case of an emergency. Give callers an option for returning to the main menu without redialing. Do not use gratuitous messages, such as "Your call is important to us," and then keep them on hold for 5 minutes. If the menu promises response to a call within a preset time, endeavor to honor that commitment.

Automated telephone systems also allow callers to access information about commonly asked questions by selecting an extension that is set up with an automated voice message. A "practice information line" can be made available on the automated attendant to handle the 1,200 calls per year that seek nonclinical, practice information. General information can be offered, such as hours of operation, directions to the practice, insurance information, hospital affiliations, and telephone care policies or instructions. This can save as much as $1,500 per year. Automated information lines also can be used to provide information about frequently asked questions ("What's going around this week?") and common illness or health information topics. Most systems provided by local telephone companies will offer at least 5 of these types of information lines for a standard office.

Voice Messaging

Voice messaging allows nonurgent calls to be batched, which allows for a more time-efficient response for nonurgent prescription refills; nonurgent nurse advice; test result inquiries; immunization questions; nonurgent business, billing, and referral issues; nonurgent messages for mid-level practitioners or physicians; and perhaps a practice suggestion mailbox. Most consumers, in general, and patients, in particular, prefer to talk to a live person rather than a machine. However, patients are not particularly pleased with waiting on the phone as it rings endlessly. Some practices will choose not to use automation because they want a more personal approach. Because there are dramatic swings in call volumes in a family practice, some combination of these 2 features might be used. During low-volume times, perhaps a person can answer the phone. During high-volume times, the automated system can be used.

Automated telephone systems allow nurses to handle batches of calls at once and then attend to other duties, rather than be continually interrupted. Voice mail systems should have prompts to guide the caller as to what information to leave for the specific type of call. Systems that allow callers to leave voice mail may be helpful but are only useful if that mail is listened to and an appropriate response is provided in a timely manner. It is very important when using a voice mail system to change the automated system messages to inform people about times when calls will go unanswered for unusually long periods.

Satisfaction rates with these systems correlate with whether the system allows the caller to speak to a person if desired. Even if you opt not to use an automated attendant, do seriously consider voice mail.

Fax

Prescriptions may account for as many as 1,000 calls per family physician per year, or as many as 50 hours of staff time. Automated telephone systems typically allow several prescription refills for an individual pharmacy to be handled with one call. Voice mail at the pharmacies for leaving multiple prescriptions also will reduce the time required. Faxing prescriptions to pharmacies that allow it can further reduce the cost. If prescription refills and health plan communication were faxed instead of handled over the phone by staff, it could save $3,000 per year per physician in the practice.

Automated Outbound Calls

Automated outbound calls can be used to confirm or remind patients about appointments. These calls may represent 14% of all calls. Office efficiency and profitability depend on high appointment "show" rates. Also, in an era of managed care and capitation, physicians will be expected to maintain and document very high immunization rates. There is a technology available that uses computer-generated telephone reminder messages to provide appointment and immunization reminders. This technology combines a computer in which names, telephone numbers, and dates are stored and an interactive voice response system with prerecorded messages on tape that is programmed to make automated reminder calls in response to the computer database. The system can complete 80 to 100 outbound telephone calls an hour and can be programmed to deliver the calls between 6:00 and 9:00 pm on weeknights, which is the most likely time to find patients available. The call can be redialed for busy signals and repeated later if there is no answer. The rate at which patients are successfully reached is approximately 70%. Computer-generated telephone reminder messages have been shown to more than double the immunization rates in 2 underserved rural populations with previously very low immunization rates. In populations with high rates of missed appointments for health supervision visits, even when immunizations are not needed, this system has improved appointment show-rates by 25%. These systems are particularly attractive to organizations that serve large populations with low immunization rates or with concerns about missed appointments; however, in populations with preexisting moderately high compliance rates, further study is needed to determine the cost benefit. When such a system is made available at no cost by a hospital, health plan, or government agency, it is worth using. However, only the very largest multispecialty groups (more than 50 physicians) will be able to afford to purchase it on their own. Outsourcing these calls to medical call centers for a fee is usually not economical.

The Internet

Internet services are increasing. Some health plans allow insurance verification and referral using Internet sites. Often, information about specialist lists and covered services are available on Web sites. Many patient education materials and medical references are available on the Internet. Internet access will soon be the norm in most practices.

E-mail

E-mail is becoming a popular means of communicating in the general public. There has been a reluctance on the part of family practitioners to open up this channel of communication with patients, originating partly from a concern that urgent issues may not be recognized quickly enough, information may not easily be secured, and from a fear that this access could be abused. However, several uses have the potential to reduce cost by reducing the time lost in making telephone connection with patients. Physician-to-physician e-mail for communication about patients, e-mail consultations, and transmission of consultation reports will improve time-efficiency. E-mailing prescriptions to pharmacies will significantly reduce staff time on the phone. Ordering tests at hospitals, ordering supplies, and communicating with health plans can be done by e-mail as well, when available. There is potential benefit in using e-mail to communicate between patients and reception/scheduling staff or the business office for appointments, health information, and nonconfidential negative test results or business issues.

Telephone Equipment

Details about selecting telephone equipment are beyond the scope of this manual. Capital expenses seem formidable, but a top-of-the-line system, when amortized over 5 years, costs between $2 and $3 a day, compared to $1 a day for the bare minimum. It is commonly recommended that a family physician's office have a minimum of 4 lines (2 incoming at the front desk and 2 outgoing in the back office). It also is commonly recommended that a minimum of 2 lines per physician in the practice be considered, up to a total of 10. Depending on the volume and complexity of insurance claims for an office, options for routine triage, dedicated administrative phone lines, and voice message mailboxes have all been employed. Because these discussions can be lengthy, complex, and, at times, contentious, it is logical to have dedicated lines, both inbound and outbound, for administrative functions. The most common complaint about the telephone service from physicians is that the lines are too often busy. Front desk lines should be sequenced so that if one line is busy, the call goes to the next line, and there should be 3 or 4 lines with people available to respond (including the office manager or business office during high-volume times). Large offices have a courtesy line for patients to use. Reception staff appreciate "hands-free" headsets, which will make them more efficient. The local telephone company normally has consultants who can make suggestions for cost-efficient ways to solve problems. The telephone system that you purchase should be able to accommodate whatever expansion plans you have for at least the next 5 years.

Chapter 20

After-Hours Telephone Care Overview

The first report in the medical literature of after-hours telephone care appeared in 1879, just 3 years after Bell invented the telephone. In that report, a general practitioner in Great Britain described listening to a child's breathing over the telephone at midnight to rule out croup and was able to prevent an after-hours house call by providing telephone advice. Physicians were the first professionals to be expected to have a telephone. Between the 1930s and 1950s there was a growing expectation that all physicians provide 24-hour telephone availability to patients. Since that time, patients' satisfaction with their physician was highly correlated with 24-hour availability of telephone advice. Although some physicians began to arrange with other physicians to occasionally cross-cover after-hours telephone calls in the 1950s, almost all physicians through the 1950s took all of their own telephone calls day and night. In the 1960s and 1970s, some physicians began to delegate office-hours clinical calls to nonphysicians. However, delegation of after-hours calls did not begin until the 1990s, and still today, family physicians take most after-hours calls to family practices in the United States. It is estimated that 20% of US family physicians delegate after-hours telephone calls to a medical call center, service bureau, or telephone triage nurse.

Although telephone care accounts for approximately 20% to 25% of all clinical care in a family practice, it accounts for as much as 80% of after-hours care. During the past quarter century, there has been an increase in

- Demand for after-hours telephone care
- Size of after-hours call groups
- Acceptance of delegating after-hours telephone care to nonphysicians
- The development of large medical call centers
- Encouragement to triage after-hours calls to the least expensive safe level of care and limit after-hours emergency department (ED) visits
- Encouragement to provide more patient education by telephone to promote self-care and appropriate use of health care resources
- Willingness to manage more chronic illnesses without a face-to-face encounter
- Medicolegal liability

As a result of these trends, the role of the family physician is expanding just as it has during office hours to include the need to understand

- Delegation of after-hours telephone care
- Selection and adaptation or approval of telephone guidelines
- Selecting, training, and evaluating telephone care providers or medical call centers
- Medicolegal risk
- Documentation
- Program (or medical call center) evaluation
- Official standards and regulations as they evolve
- Effects of managed care and capitation on after-hours telephone care

Demographics of After-Hours Telephone Care

The number of after-hours calls to a family physician over the course of a year varies dramatically from practice to practice and even by region of the country. The average number of after-hours calls to a family physician appears to be between 500 and 1,000 per year, with a mean of around 700 calls per year per physician in the practice. Ninety percent of these calls are clinical and the rest administrative (eg, prescription refills, authorizing ED visits, dealing with insurance issues). On average, family physicians handle 1 to 2 calls per weeknight per physician in the practice and 2 to 3 calls per weekend day and night per physician, varying with the size of the practice, age of the patient population, and time of year. The after-hours summer call volume is between 65% and 70% of the winter call volume. Between 40% and 45% of after-hours calls are made between 5:00 and 11:00 pm Monday through Friday; between 40% and 45% are made between 8:00 am and 11:00 pm Saturday and Sunday; and 10% of calls occur between 11:00 pm and 8:00 am, 7 days per week. There are 119 to 123 "after hours" (hours when the office is not open) in a week, depending on whether the practice is open on Saturday mornings. For most family practices, 85% to 90% of after-hours calls come in during the 60 "peak after hours" (5:00–11:00 pm on weeknights and 8:00 am–11:00 pm on weekends). The remaining 10% to 15% of calls come in during the 63 overnight, "nonpeak hours" (11:00 pm–8:00 am).

Because family practices vary in patient population age distribution and their individual interests in obstetric, pediatric, and geriatric care, call distributions vary widely. Family practices that provide the entire spectrum of care have call distributions as shown in Table 20-1. Table 20-2 lists the 20 most frequent reasons for after-hours calls to a family practice.

The following patient characteristics are associated with a higher frequency of telephone calls to physicians: either very young or very old patient age, less knowledge of health care, increased socioeconomic status, and socially isolated patients. Between 10% and 20% of calls are judged by the on-call physician to be unnecessary. The seriousness and necessity of the calls do not increase after midnight.

Managing After-Hours Telephone Care

Physician Perceptions of After-Hours Telephone Care

The first cautionary letter to the editor about the risk of patients abusing telephone access to physicians was written in 1883, and an ambivalence among physicians about the telephone has been apparent in the literature ever since. Family physicians have perceived the telephone as one of the greatest sources of pressure in office practice and after-hours care.

Delegating Telephone Care to Nonphysicians

During the late 1980s, some physicians began to delegate after-hours telephone calls to non-physicians, although there is little documentation in the literature until the 1990s when community-wide nurse triage and advice services began to emerge. Although most private practice family physicians in the United States still handle their after-hours calls, in large cities a growing number of physicians delegate at least some of their after-hours telephone calls. The rationale for delegating after-hours telephone care to nonphysicians includes reduced physician stress and burnout, improved physician performance during office hours, improved documentation, and standardization of care. Patient satisfaction with delegating after-hours calls also has been high (94%-98%).

Table 20-1 After-Hours Telephone Call Demographics for a Family Practice That Provides Obstetric, Pediatric, and Geriatric Patient Care	
Type of Caller	**Percentage of Calls**
Patient or family member	66
Hospital	15
Nursing home	5
Emergency department	10
Pharmacy	3
Other	1
Age of Patient (Years)	**Percentage of Calls**
0-14	33
15-21	10
22-44	40
45-64	10
65 and older	7
Disposition of Call	**Percentage of Calls**
Telephone advice only	60-70
Call in prescription	5-15
Sent to emergency department	10-20
Appointment during next available office hours	5-15
Hospitalize	1-5
Type of Problem	**Percentage of Calls**
Medical	60-75
Trauma	15-20
Obstetric	3-6
Psychosocial	2-5
Prescription related	5-10
Day of Week	**Percentage of Calls**
Monday	10
Tuesday	9
Wednesday	9
Thursday	9
Friday	10
Saturday	25
Sunday	28

Table 20-2 After-Hours Telephone Calls to Family Physicians—Top Symptoms	
Symptom	**Percentage of All After-Hours Calls**
1. Trauma, injury	17
2. Fever	10
3. Medication questions	7
4. Obstetric	8
5. Upper respiratory infection	5
6. Nausea, vomiting	5
7. Asthma	4
8. Abdominal pain	8
9. Chest pain	3
10. Eye symptoms	2
11. Rash	4
12. Cough	4
13. Back pain	3
14. Headache	3
15. Sore throat	3
16. Ear symptoms	3
17. Laboratory test results	3
18. Diarrhea	2
19. Anxiety	2
20. Diabetes	2

Comparing Providers

There are no comprehensive studies comparing outcomes of after-hours calls taken by physicians with registered nurses (RNs) using after-hours telephone care guidelines. Nor are there comparisons among mid-level practitioners, RNs, licensed practical nurses, or medical assistants. However, after-hours telephone care is more difficult and a higher risk than telephone care during office hours, and there is a consensus that it should be delegated to someone with at least RN training.

Training

The training of nurses to provide after-hours telephone care should proceed as described in Chapter 6. Only the most experienced and accomplished should be assigned to provide after-hours coverage.

Medicolegal Issues Associated With Managed Care

In addition to the already substantial liability associated with telephone care in general, managed care adds the considerable additional associated risk with its objectives to limit access to care and direct patients to lower-cost providers and facilities. A backlash is forming in response to what the public perceives as limitation of care. Juries have shown clearly their disapproval of attempts to use the telephone to cut costs if there is a bad outcome. The Colorado Division of Insurance (like most other states) has recently instituted new regulations requiring health plans to pay for emergency care or urgent care for any condition that could be perceived by a reasonable layperson to be an urgent medical need, even if the primary care provider does not perceive the need to be urgent. It is acceptable, under these regulations, to make recommendations to callers about self-care or selection of a site of care, but physicians have less authority to manage care by telephone even though health plans provide incentives to do so. Therefore, telephone triage must be relatively conservative at the present time and should focus on quality care, patient satisfaction, and appropriate resource use without taking undue chances. For more information, see Chapter 2.

Documentation

Although careful documentation is one of the most important means of reducing liability in telephone care, fewer than half of physicians document after-hours telephone calls. Good documentation of telephone calls also enhances other practice functions: medical record keeping, continuity of care, complaint resolution, patient care follow-up, and quality assurance. Medicolegally, all after-hours calls that involve any clinical decision making or advice should be documented in the manner described in Chapter 4.

After-Hours Telephone Triage and Advice Guidelines

Health care professionals make potentially serious mistakes when they do not use telephone care guidelines. Skills, performance, and behavior in telephone care vary greatly, and training in telephone care for all types of providers has been limited. The length of experience or level of training does not correlate with performance in handling test scenarios or simulations. Documentation is often neglected, and even when documentation exists, it often is not adequate. Health plans are under increasing pressure to standardize care provided by contracted physicians. Poor physician performance on standardized tests of telephone care skills relates to lack of a consistent, organized approach. Guidelines have been shown to be safe, effective, and acceptable to patients and physicians; reduce the medicolegal risk of telephone care by improving documentation and standardizing care; and improve documentation by reducing the time required for complete documentation. At least one major medical malpractice carrier gives a premium discount to practices that regularly use telephone guidelines for after-hours care. For these reasons, it is recommended that after-hours telephone triage and advice, no matter who is providing them, follow established telephone decision-making guidelines. If experienced physicians decide not to carry telephone care guidelines with them while on call, they should at least require nurses who do after-hours telephone triage and advice and physicians who are new to practice to use them.

The dispositions for after-hours telephone triage and advice are different from those used in the office during the day. If office-hours guidelines are going to be used for after-hours coverage, be sure to review them and adapt the dispositions for after-hours care. It is possible to purchase specific after-hours telephone care guidelines for pediatric telephone care, such as *Pediatric Telephone Protocols: After-Hours Version*, 9th Edition, by Barton D. Schmitt, MD.

Telephone Triage and Advice by Nonphysicians in Managed Care

In a fee-for-service era, families that wanted an appointment during office hours usually received one, and families who wanted to go to an ED after hours did so. For managed care populations, there are incentives for providers to rigorously triage after-hours telephone calls. For capitated populations, physicians will benefit from subjecting all illness calls 24 hours a day to a telephone triage process. Physicians who are in the position of needing to carefully manage after-hours use of health care resources should be aware that a nurse using telephone care guidelines refers about twice as many patients for after-hours medical care than physicians do. Nurses using guidelines to provide after-hours telephone care manage 70% of calls without an after-hours visit by recommending self-care (50%) or an appointment during regular office hours (20%). That means that 30% are directed to seek after-hours emergent or urgent care. Family physicians can manage 80% to 90% of calls without an after-hours visit. The reasons that physicians are more able than nurses to triage patients away from after-hours emergency care include (1) greater comfort with managing a higher level of illness than the nurse, (2) prior knowledge of the family's ability to assess or care for the patient, (3) greater willingness to provide interim advice and call the patient back, and (4) prior knowledge of the patient's medical history. Physicians also more often manage calls without an after-hours visit by advising callers to visit the office early the next day.

Therefore, when after-hours telephone care is delegated to nurses for a managed care or capitated population, physicians should consider using 2 levels of triage: (1) a nurse using guidelines to respond to all calls and (2) a physician to take those 30% of calls that the nurse and guidelines identify as possibly needing after-hours care. The physician can reduce the number of ED referrals from 30% to 10% or 20%.

Medical Call Centers and Service Bureaus

Medical call centers are large-scale telephone triage and advice programs provided, usually by hospitals, on a local basis for physicians. Service bureaus are for-profit companies providing large-scale telephone care services covering wide areas, usually serving health plans or large health care organizations. These 2 alternatives are described in Chapter 21.

Answering Services

Between 90% and 98% of family physicians use an answering service. And, although answering service personnel receive no training in clinical triage, they often perform triage and advice functions. A survey of physicians and their answering services in the 1980s revealed considerable discrepancies between what the physician authorized the answering service personnel to do and what they actually did: (1) 3.5% of physicians authorized their answering service to give advice to callers, but the answering services gave advice of a clinical nature to the callers on behalf of 20% of physicians; (2) 3% of physicians authorized their answering service to relay prescription requests to pharmacies, but the services performed this function on behalf of 35% of physicians; and (3) 15% of answering services referred patients to EDs without authorization. Answering service personnel can be an untrained and unauthorized source of telephone triage and advice in family practice and warrant close scrutiny. Family physicians should clearly communicate to their answering service the limits of what it is authorized to do, and physicians should periodically use mock calls to corroborate that the service is performing as expected. Also, just as documentation is a very important element of telephone care for the clinician, a major criterion for selecting an answering service should be the service's ability to thoroughly document and retain information on all calls.

After-Hours Care and Emergency Departments

Approximately 60% of visits to an ED are judged unnecessary. Factors associated with higher ED use include the patient's perception of higher severity of illness, stress, lower socioeconomic status, and, most importantly, lack of availability of telephone advice.

Telephone Care by Emergency Departments

Most community hospital EDs receive between 25 and 50 telephone calls for medical advice each day. The telephone advice provided by hospital EDs varies widely, usually is not based on telephone care protocols or accepted policies and procedures, usually averages less than 2 minutes per call, and often provides inadequate assessment. In 45% of urgent care centers, receptionists gave the telephone advice, and 83% of urgent care center advice was judged inadequate. Because medicolegal liability is high when dealing with strangers over the phone, and because EDs do not have a legal duty to treat unless and until they begin to offer advice, many EDs have been advised by legal counsel, the American College of Emergency Physicians, and emergency nurse professional organizations not to give advice, but instead recommend that patients come in for care. Nearly 90% of callers to an ED are advised to come in to be seen, compared with 20% of after-hours callers to physicians being told to go in for care. When EDs establish a telephone nurse triage line, between 20% to 55% of patients are directed to come in for care. In summary, EDs are greatly overused for health care and the current trend in EDs to avoid giving telephone advice promotes further overuse of the EDs. However, an organized approach to nurse triage by the ED can significantly reduce the proportion of unnecessary visits. It is not wise to "sign out" (turn over after-hours telephone calls) to the ED, as was done by some physicians in previous decades, unless the ED has developed a system like the hospital medical call centers described in Chapter 21.

Reimbursement

Reimbursement for after-hours telephone care is favored by 90% of physicians. *Current Procedural Terminology (CPT)* codes for the telephone care of ill or injured patients exist for calls handled by physicians. There are no *CPT* codes for telephone care provided by nurses. Few physicians charge for telephone care, but a recent study suggests that reimbursement, when pursued, can be obtained from many health plans (but not from Medicaid or Medicare yet). Billing health plans for those after-hours calls handled by physicians is recommended. A survey of physicians suggested charging $20 for brief calls (**99371**); $30 for calls about a new acute problem (**99372**); and $50 when a complex, time-consuming problem is handled after hours (**99373**). (See Chapter 16.)

Coverage Options

In many large cities there are a variety of options for coverage of after-hours telephone care.

- Physician on call
- Mid-level practitioner on call
- Nurse on call
- Medical call center
- Service bureau
- Combinations

The next 3 chapters describe these options and provide guidelines for selecting among them.

Physician Coverage

Physicians have provided after-hours telephone triage and advice for generations. With the increasing volume, complexity, medicolegal risk, and resultant stress associated with after-hours telephone care, many physicians are reevaluating how they provide this important service. Most are looking for help in handling after-hours calls, and many are open to suggestions on changing how they manage telephone care when they are on call. A few points can be made here about physicians taking their own after-hours telephone calls.

Most family physicians do not receive much formal training in telephone care. They learn on the job. The use of telephone care guidelines improves and shortens the learning process for residents and new physicians. Therefore, at least during training and in the early years in practice, physicians should consider using telephone care guidelines. Telephone care guidelines reduce medicolegal risk, improve standardization of care within a practice, provide continuing education, make documentation easier and quicker, improve the quality of documentation, and improve quality of care. In addition, family physicians have to respond to a much broader array of clinical conditions over the phone than any other specialty. So, all family physicians should think about keeping these guidelines available while on call. Family physicians who take their own night calls often carry with them a "peripheral brain," a notebook with key phone numbers, difficult to remember dosages, clinical protocols, and managed care referral information. We recommend considering adding telephone care guidelines to that peripheral brain. Using standardized, accepted telephone care guidelines and documenting each clinical call can protect a family physician against telephone care malpractice allegations.

Chapter 21

Medical Call Centers and Service Bureaus

Medical call centers are telephone care programs that employ nurses who use telephone care guidelines to provide telephone triage and advice and health information. They are usually run by, and based in, community or children's hospitals and serve local physicians. Service bureaus are for-profit companies providing large-scale telephone care services over wide geographic areas, usually serving health plans or large health care organizations. Medical call centers and service bureaus also may provide other telephone services, such as physician finding and referral, appointment scheduling for offices, answering services, and general health information on common topics for the general public. Medical call centers are best known to physicians for their after-hours telephone triage and advice service.

Medical Call Centers

In the 1990s, large medical call centers were started by hospitals or health maintenance organizations to encourage physician allegiance, improve physician quality of life, and better manage access to care. Medical call centers are staffed by nurses using telephone care guidelines and provide telephone triage and advice for patients or their parents from local or affiliated practices. Currently in the United States, approximately 400 general hospitals or health plans operate medical call centers that provide telephone care. It is estimated that 20% of family physicians were using a medical call center in 1999. Medical call centers most often purchase a software product from a for-profit company that incorporates telephone care guidelines into an automated documentation system. Most medical call centers employ nurses from a variety of specialties.

Medical call centers provided by hospitals have shown high levels of caller satisfaction (94%-98%) and physician satisfaction (98%-100%). Patient compliance with nurse triage and advice has been between 90% and 95%. Complaint rates are in the range of 1%. Currently there are no published data that examine clinical outcomes of patients managed by medical call centers. It is clear, however, that there is a high level of concordance between physicians and the dispositions and advice provided by these medical call centers. Studies have shown that in a fee-for-service system, 40% to 70% of after-hours calls to a medical call center are managed without an after-hours health care visit. Physicians agree with this disposition 70% to 80% of the time.

Comparing Telephone Care by Medical Call Centers With Telephone Care by Physicians

The benefits of a well-managed medical call center compared with a physician on call include better documentation, better standardization of care, more teaching for the caller, reduced medicolegal risk for the practice, the ability to review statistical data from after-hours calls, and improved lifestyle for the physician. The disadvantages are greater expense to the health care system and decreased managed care capability. Table 21-1 presents information from health care literature of the past 10 years and compares medical call centers with primary care physicians.

Table 21-1 Comparison of Telephone Care Provided by Medical Call Centers Versus Physicians		
	Medical Call Centers	**Physicians**
Average call length	7-10 minutes	3-4 minutes
Compliance by caller	85%	95%
Percentage of all calls referred to an after-hours emergency department or urgent care center	25%-50%	10%-20%
Caller satisfaction	94%-98%	94%-96%

Financial Status of Medical Call Centers

The average expense per call handled by medical call centers is between $12 and $20, but the reimbursement from the physicians for whom the care is provided ranges from $0 to $15. Therefore, general hospitals that provide medical call centers for their referring physicians usually run large deficits. Many hospital administrators accept those deficits because the programs create high degrees of patient and physician allegiance and satisfaction. However, in recent years, hospitals have been less able to afford to so heavily subsidize these programs and some have closed. Even if hospitals wanted to continue to subsidize, they are limited in terms of how much they can subsidize. Federal regulations do not allow hospitals to provide a service to doctors at less than fair market value. Therefore, many of the hospitals that continue to sponsor medical call centers are significantly increasing their charges. Physicians who have previously used medical call centers are finding themselves unable to find coverage or afford the coverage they had. Ways in which physicians can adapt to this situation are described in chapters 22 and 23.

Why Medical Call Centers Are More Expensive

There are several reasons why medical call centers cost more than office-based telephone nurse triage, including higher nursing salaries and benefits, additional after-hours salary differentials, a higher level of training for telephone nurse providers (often bachelor's level registered nurses [RNs]), more attention to quality assurance and risk reduction (eg, audits, audiotaping calls, better documentation), software with automated documentation (more expensive and time-consuming), higher overhead expenses, staffing costs during low-volume times (including high hourly premiums to allow flexible staffing for giant swings in volume), more supervision, and longer and more extensive training for nurses.

The reasons that medical call centers are more expensive are, in most instances, well worth it when they are available to a physician. Having an after-hours telephone triage and advice program in your practice that you control and that costs less than many medical call centers charge may be appealing. However, there is more to the decision to start your own program than just economic considerations. To match the quality of clinical care and the low medi-colegal risk found in a medical call center, the physician or trusted designee will be required to spend a great deal of time and energy attending to issues such as recruitment, staffing, adapting schedules to the dramatic swings in call volume, reducing medicolegal risk, training staff, reviewing telephone call logs, monitoring quality assurance issues, developing policies, completing performance evaluations, and organizing call flow. For those physicians who are currently using a medical call center, most will be willing to pay the difference between what the medical call center charges and the cost of setting up their own program to obtain high-quality coverage for their patients and avoid extra demands on their professional time. For those practices without access to a good, affordable medical call center, the next chapter describes how to create an after-hours telephone triage and advice program to cover the practice.

Service Bureaus

Over the past 10 to 15 years, for-profit companies with marketing, rather than medical, backgrounds have developed regional telephone triage and advice call centers called "service bureaus." They served mostly health plans or hospital systems initially, although a few are providing services to practices now. Because they are for-profit, their charges range from $15 to $25 per call. Service bureaus usually serve large health care organizations that can afford such high prices. They tend to refer a higher proportion of patients for after-hours care than medical call centers. So the disadvantages of service bureaus include expense and high rates of after-hours referral for care. At the present time service bureaus are not recommended. However, physicians without access to a medical call center, but who have an option to use a service bureau, should carefully assess the service bureau using the same criteria as in evaluating a medical call center. (See following text.)

Quality and Assessment

Quality

Until recently there have been no national standards and no official organizations with authority to regulate or accredit either service bureaus or medical call centers. The American Accreditation Health Care Commission/URAC (a nonprofit organization created to develop standards for the health care industry and promote high quality for its member organizations) accredits managed care organizations. Voluntary accreditation is available for medical call centers that provide 24-hour-a-day telephone triage. The American Academy of Pediatrics Section on Telephone Care, working with the American Association of Ambulatory Care Nursing, proposed standards (expectations) for medical call centers. A copy of these recommendations is included in Appendix C. National standards of care, regulation, and accreditation are needed for all types of medical call centers.

Assessment of Medical Call Centers

Physicians, before entrusting their patients to a medical call center or service bureau, should carefully assess the quality of the guidelines, credentials of the nurses and medical director, training and supervision of the nurses, quality assurance process, availability of physicians to backup or answer questions for the nurses, and completeness of documentation. Also, because most medical call centers are unable to sustain themselves without subsidy at the present time, the subscribing physician should understand the underlying objectives of the subsidizing organization. Other outcome measures that the physician should check include

- Call response time
- Call duration
- Caller satisfaction rates
- Physician satisfaction rates
- Complaint rate
- Call disposition rates (ie, percent of calls referred for after-hours care, office appointment the next day, and self-care)
- Percentage of calls reviewed for quality improvement

The preferred medical call center is one that is run locally, seeks plenty of input from local physicians, has a local physician as medical director, allows guidelines to be customized to local standards of care, provides complete documentation of all calls, is overseen by a medical advisory committee made up of local physicians, employs well-trained and experienced RNs, maintains policies and procedures governing at least the issues covered in Chapter 9, has a quality assurance program, responds quickly to emergencies, and provides you with documentation of urgent after-hours calls by the next morning. It is wise, as well, to test the medical call center by calling it yourself, posing as a patient seeking advice.

Effective Use of Medical Call Centers

Be sure that you provide instructions for your answering service (or on the office's after-hours automated attendant message) to limit the calls to the medical call center to only those truly requiring after-hours triage and advice or urgent health information. Calls for nonclinical information, nonurgent refills, appointments, and so on should be postponed until the next office hours to limit the number of calls for which you are charged.

Some family physicians, for the reasons described previously, find themselves unable to afford medical call center coverage of all of the after-hours calls that come to their practice. The most important principle in dealing with medical call center prices that are too expensive is to recognize the peak volume hours during which after-hours clinical telephone calls come into the practice and find a less expensive way to handle those calls (Chapter 23). This can be accomplished by combining medical call center coverage with other options for after-hours telephone care coverage. For example, the physician may take his or her own calls until 11:00 pm and have the medical call center take calls after that. In this way, the physician pays the medical call center only for handling the 10% to 15% of the after-hours calls that occur after 11:00 pm. Another option is to create an after-hours nurse triage system using nurses within the practice to manage the after-hours calls. This usually can be done during peak after hours for $4 to $6 a call. When this option is used for peak after hours, the remaining 10% to 15% of calls can be handled either by the physician or practice nurses (while being paid at a higher rate to accommodate the after-hours nature of their work) or the medical call center. Chapter 23 describes the various combinations in detail.

Some medical call centers or service bureaus offer an answering service as a companion program. If you use both services, you may receive the answering service at a lower rate than you might pay for an answering service alone. They can do this because they are able to take advantage of economies of scale by combining staffs, equipment, etc. This may allow you to obtain the combination of answering service and medical call center for a reasonable combined price.

Medical Call Centers and Managed Care (Second-Level Triage)

As described in the previous chapter, telephone triage and advice nurses, using very good telephone triage and advice guidelines, are able to manage 50% to 70% of after-hours calls without an after-hours visit. A physician, however, can manage 80% to 90% without an after-hours visit, particularly in a managed care environment. When a physician signs out to a medical call center, there is the potential for many more patients to be directed in for care than if the physician was taking the calls. In an unmanaged health care system, most physicians feel this is a small price to pay for the improvement in the quality of their on-call existence. In a managed care environment, this trade-off may not seem worth it. In that case, a second-level physician triage is recommended. Calls are taken by the medical call center, but when the medical call center nurse, using the telephone care guidelines, feels the patient should be seen after hours, the call is directed back to the physician instead of telling the patient to be seen after hours. This gives the physician a chance to put the patient through a second triage and reduce the number of patients actually sent in for after-hours care. In this way, the physician takes only 30% of the total after-hours calls but maintains the same level of managed care.

Chapter 22

An After-Hours Telephone Nurse Triage System Using Office Nurses

Most family physicians describe after-hours telephone care as one of the most frustrating and stressful aspects of practice. Delegating after-hours telephone care began in the 1990s. Now 20% of after-hours calls in the United States are being taken by telephone triage nurses in medical call centers. Many family physicians who have not delegated after-hours calls wish to do so; however, many medical call centers managed by general hospitals are experiencing financial difficulties. Some are closing and many must charge more than family physicians can afford. The after-hours telephone triage provided by for-profit service bureaus usually charge more than family physicians can afford. In addition, most family physicians practice in areas that do not have access to a call center of any kind. Many of these physicians consider developing their own after-hours call center within their practice.

Chapter 21 describes the many reasons to use a medical call center if one is available and affordable. For those practices without access to an affordable medical call center, this chapter describes how to create an office-based, after-hours telephone triage and advice program.

Delegating After-Hours Telephone Care
Delegating after-hours telephone care is well accepted by patients. There are studies and reports that suggest nursing training improves the performance of someone who provides telephone triage and advice. There are no studies to tell us what minimum acceptable level of nursing training is required for after-hours telephone care. However, nearly all medical call centers require a registered nurse (RN) degree. After-hours telephone care nurses should be selected from among those nurses who have proven themselves to be very competent in providing telephone care during office hours.

Medicolegal Risk
Juries in telephone malpractice cases have indicated that delegation of after-hours care to nurses is acceptable as long as they have been trained, use standardized guidelines, document their calls, have physician backup, and are regularly evaluated. To prove malpractice, a plaintiff must prove care did not meet community standards. If the nurse follows standardized, accepted guidelines and adequately documents a call, it is difficult to prove malpractice. Therefore, the 2 most important risk reduction methods are (1) following standardized telephone guidelines in an exact manner and (2) documenting the triage and advice completely. To our knowledge, there have been no after-hours telephone care malpractice judgments against an after-hours telephone care system when the triage nurse followed standardized after-hours telephone triage and advice guidelines and completely documented the call. Another important way to reduce medicolegal risks is to allow patients to be seen if they do not feel comfortable with home care instructions.

Telephone Care Guidelines

Telephone care guidelines provide standardization of care and make documentation easier and faster. Because developing guidelines is very time-consuming and wide acceptance of the guidelines reduces medicolegal risk, it is wise to purchase guidelines rather than develop your own. However, you will have to review and adapt them (particularly the symptomatic treatment) to ensure that they are consistent with your practice's style. Also, be sure that the dispositions are consistent with your practice style and fit the options for after-hours care in your community. Be sure that the guidelines cover at least 100 symptoms, have been tested in clinical settings, and were written for after-hours use or have been adapted for appropriate after-hours dispositions. This requires that a physician in your practice review the guidelines. The most difficult step in the triage and advice process is selecting the appropriate symptom guideline. Be sure that the guidelines you select provide guidance on guideline selection. There are at least 4 sets of guidelines that meet these criteria.

- Brown JL. *Pediatric Telephone Medicine: Principles, Triage, and Advice.* 2nd ed. Philadelphia, PA: Lippincott Williams & Wilkins; 1994
- Katz HP. *Telephone Medicine: Triage and Training for Primary Care.* 2nd ed. Philadelphia, PA: F. A. Davis Co; 2001
- Schmitt BD. *Pediatric Telephone Protocols: After-Hours Version.* 9th ed. Littleton, CO: Decision Press; 2002
- Thompson DA. *Adult Telephone Protocols: After-Hours Version.* Littleton, CO: Decision Press; 2003

Avoid triage and advice software because it can add at least 2 minutes to the after-hours call and it is usually more expensive than most groups of family physicians (fewer than 50) can afford.

Documentation

Documentation of all after-hours calls that involve triage or any type of advice is imperative. Written telephone logs using efficient checklists are preferred. Nurses can abbreviate documentation by indicating the guideline used, indicating only the positive responses to questions from the guidelines, and writing "advice per guideline." Minimal documentation for clinical calls includes caller name, relationship to patient, phone number, patient name and age, date and time, reason for call, guideline used, pertinent positives on history, disposition, summary of advice (can write "per guideline"), dosages (can write "per guideline"), caller acceptance of advice, callback instructions (can write "per guideline"), and signature. (See sample logs in Chapter 4.) From a medicolegal standpoint, documentation of clinical calls should be retrievable. A dictated or written note in the patient chart is the best documentation, but documentation can be retained in separate telephone call logbooks. Telephone logs from the previous night should be given to the primary care physician to review at the beginning of each day.

A Cost-efficient After-Hours Nurse Triage System

The cost-efficiency of an after-hours coverage system using telephone triage nurses depends mostly on call duration, the number of calls per hour that the nurse can handle, scheduling of the nurse, and creative approaches for compensating the telephone triage nurse.

Call Duration

Call duration should reflect a balance between quality of care and caller satisfaction on one hand and efficient methods on the other. Nurse training, described in Chapter 6, is very important for quality of care, caller satisfaction, and cost-efficiency. Describing the model call and target call duration is the key step. (See Chapter 6.) Establishing standards of performance for how to handle each component of the call and the duration of each component also is important. After-hours telephone triage and advice calls may take longer than office-hours clinical calls because fewer patients are directed to see a provider, more triage is needed, and often more advice is given to tide the patient overnight. Also, fewer of the calls are for health information only. In addition, there is an average of $1\frac{1}{2}$ calls per after-hours telephone case because the nurse may need to call a pharmacy, refer the patient to an emergency department (ED), or check with the physician. A target call duration for triage and advice should be no more than 7 to 8 minutes, unless another call is needed to complete the case. The target for health information-only calls is still 3 to 4 minutes, but the nurse needs to be sure that triage is not needed.

Staffing

Understanding your call demographics is a first step in deciding what hours to delegate to a telephone triage nurse and how to staff those hours. There are between 119 and 123 after hours (hours when the office is not open) in a week, depending on whether the practice is open on Saturday mornings. For most practices, 85% to 90% of after-hours calls come in during the 60 peak after hours (weeknights 5:00-11:00 pm and weekends 8:00 am-11:00 pm). The remaining 10% to 15% of calls come in during the 63 overnight, nonpeak hours (11:00 pm-8:00 am). Acuity is not higher among nonpeak calls than peak-time calls. The actual volume of calls varies with the season. The lowest summer volumes usually are 65% of the highest winter volumes. There also is a great variation among practices because of practice styles. Therefore, each practice should collect its own after-hours call volume data to use for planning. One family physician generates between 500 and 1,000 after-hours calls per year. In Colorado, family physicians average 11 after-hours calls per week per physician in the practice in the summer (1 per weeknight and 3 per weekend day and night per physician) and 16 calls per week per physician in the winter (1-2 per weeknight, 4 per weekend day and night per physician). See Table 22-1 for data on after-hours call volumes from a study of family practices in Colorado.

Scheduling

Scheduling telephone triage nurses to adequately cover the peak demands and avoid the overstaffing of low-volume periods is a difficult challenge. To plan, consider the number of calls per hour the triage nurse can handle and the hourly call volume (estimates are provided, but you should gather your own data). An experienced nurse using telephone care guidelines and time-efficient, written documentation logs should be able to handle 7 to 10 telephone cases an hour (6-8 minutes per triage call plus breaks). Table 22-2 shows the number of family physicians in Colorado that an experienced, trained, efficient triage nurse (with written, efficient documentation and after-hours triage and advice guidelines) can cover during various times of the week, both summer and winter.

Table 22-1 Summary of After-Hours Call Volumes for Family Practices in Colorado		
Hours of Coverage	**Average Number of Calls per Full-time Family Physician (Summer)**	**Average Number of Calls per Full-time Family Physician (Winter)**
Weeknights 5:00–11:00 pm 11:00 pm–8:00 am	1 (5/week) 0.1	1-2 (8/week) 0.3
Saturday 12:00 noon–11:00 pm 11:00 pm–8:00 am	3 0.2	4 0.3
Sunday 8:00 am–11:00 pm 11:00 pm–8:00 am	3 0.34	4 0.4
Average per week	11	16

Based on these data, then, it is estimated that one nurse can cover peak hours for 25 to 35 family physicians (depending on the season), when the call volumes and distribution are similar to that found in a study of Colorado family practices. The most efficient system is one that serves between 25 and 30 family physicians, or multiples of 25 physicians. Therefore, a practice can combine resources with other family practices to create an after-hours call coverage system.

The location of the nurse while performing telephone triage can be either at the office or at home. From a patient care standpoint, taking calls from the office is best to access medical records for patients with chronic problems or recent, ongoing acute problems. Nurse satisfaction is higher when working from home, especially during low-volume times. The nurse will be most efficient if she does not have to respond to direct calls, but instead receives calls on a voice messaging system or through an answering service. This allows the nurse to prioritize the calls.

Compensation

Compensating after-hours telephone triage nurses can be done either on an hourly basis or on a per-call basis. Because all of the other telephone expenses are fixed expenses, nurse compensation for after-hours telephone care is essentially the only significant incremental expense for this system. Because the range of hourly compensation for office RNs is so broad across the United States ($13-$30 per hour), decisions about compensation must be made based on local data. It seems fair to pay an after-hours premium. The tradition is to pay a $2 to $3 differential or 15% to 20% above the regular hourly compensation. Paying on an hourly basis is cost-effective when the nurse is busy. However, when the nurse is covering for a small number of physicians or covering a low-volume time, it is more economical to pay on a per-call basis.

	Table 22-2 **Number of Family Physicians Covered by One Telephone Care Provider During** **Different After-Hour Periods and Seasons**	
Hours of Coverage	**Number of Family Physicians One Telephone Care Provider Can Cover (Summer)**	**Number of Family Physicians One Telephone Care Provider Can Cover (Winter)**
Weeknights		
5:00–11:00 pm	35	25
11:00 pm–1:00 am	60	45
1:00–6:00 am	300	200
6:00–8:00 am	200	150
Weekends		
8:00 am–12:00 noon	35	25
12:00 noon–11:00 pm	40	25
11:00 pm–1:00 am	60	45
1:00–6:00 am	300	200
6:00–8:00 am	200	150

Calculation of the per-call compensation rate begins by determining a comfortable number of calls per hour during a moderately busy time that would promote good telephone care, a high level of caller satisfaction, and a break for the telephone triage nurse each hour. You might choose 7-minute calls at 8 calls per hour. Remember, calls for health information only usually take 4 minutes. The per-call compensation rate can be determined by calculating

$$\frac{\text{regular hourly salary} + \text{benefits} + \text{after-hours differential pay}}{\text{calls per hour}}$$

In Denver, CO, family practices the calculation might be

$$\frac{\$16 \text{ (hourly pay)} + \$3.50 \text{ (benefits)} + \$3.20 \text{ (20\% after-hours premium)}}{7 \text{ calls}} = \$3.25/\text{call}$$

When the nurse is working at a comfortable pace with only a 5-minute break per hour, she will make roughly the same pay whether paid hourly or per call. If your nursing staff is resistant to compensation on a per-call basis or does not feel this is fair, you may consider adding $0.50 to $1 per call. This allows the nurse to earn more during high-volume times and still allows the practice to contain costs during low-volume times. This also is significantly less than most medical call centers charge.

In a practice in which office nurses earn more than $16 per hour, the compensation would be proportionally higher. If you ask the nurse to handle calls during late-night or early-morning times, $3 to $4 a call may not seem fair and the rate should be increased. When a nurse is scheduled to cover a block of time during which it is anticipated that she will be earning significantly less if paid by the call compared to being paid by the hour, she should receive a guaranteed minimum hourly or shift pay (perhaps 25%-40% of normal hourly pay).

The affordability of having a nurse from the practice handle after-hours telephone care depends on having enough work for the nurse if she is paid on an hourly basis. For example, in a 5-physician family practice, if telephone triage nurses are paid on an hourly basis, the cost per call for the practice during the hours of 5:00 to 11:00 pm in the summer would be more than $10 per call. For a 25-physician call group, on average, the cost per call would be approximately $4 per call. If the nurse covers 15 physicians during nonpeak hours and is paid on an hourly basis, the cost per call would be in the range of $30 to $40 per call. For groups of fewer than 20 to 25 physicians, compensation on a per-call basis, even for peak times, is usually more cost-effective than an hourly rate. And for low-volume times, per-call compensation is nearly always more cost-effective. One option is to pay on an hourly basis during peak hours and on a per-call basis during nonpeak hours. Another option is to set up a telephone triage nurse system in your office for peak after hours and have the on-call physician cover the nonpeak hours.

Training
Training of the telephone triage nurse is described in Chapter 6. Performance evaluation is described in Chapter 7. Training should occur during office hours, and only the most experienced nurses should provide after-hours telephone care. As mentioned in Chapter 3, the most difficult step for nurses is symptom guideline selection. The physician who supervises the after-hours telephone triage nurse should carefully review with the nurse strategies for selecting the appropriate symptom guideline and review common scenarios.

Standards
Standards have been proposed for medical call centers by the American Association of Ambulatory Care Nursing and the American Academy of Pediatrics Section on Pediatric Telephone Care and Committee on Practice and Ambulatory Medicine (Appendix C). At present, practices are not held to these standards by accrediting bodies or case law. However, over time this may occur. In the meantime, these standards provide a target. As a private practice develops performance standards for its telephone triage nurses, it should review the standards for medical call centers.

A physician or mid-level practitioner in the practice should serve as medical director for after-hours telephone care and oversee the establishment of expectations and standards. Standards may include an average call duration equal to or less than 8 minutes, a rate of following telephone guidelines of 100%, a documentation rate of 100%, a caller satisfaction rate of 95%, a caller complaint rate of less than 1%, evidence that all policies are followed, a target callback time within 30 minutes, and so on. (See Chapter 7.) Standards should be tracked using periodic audits. (See Chapter 14.)

Written after-hours telephone care policies, which supplement the telephone triage and advice guidelines, ensure that care is rendered in a fashion that reflects your practice style. Ultimately, the family physician should decide the specifics of the policies, although samples are provided in Chapter 9. Policies should include how to prioritize and sequence calls; how to handle patients who demand to speak to the physician; in which conditions and situations the nurse can call in prescriptions without talking to the physician; which situations (in addition to being directed by the guidelines) in which the nurse should call the physician;

how to handle calls from minors, non–English-speaking callers, repeat callers, or callers who are not related to the patient; how to respond when callers disagree with advice; how to handle calls about abuse or neglect; and how to respond to busy lines, voice messaging, and no-answer calls.

In a managed care environment, in which there are incentives for limiting after-hours emergency visits, the physician will want to participate in all decisions involving referral to an ED. A telephone triage nurse, using telephone guidelines, will handle 50% to 70% of calls with home care instructions only and 10% to 20% of calls with home care until the next available appointment during regular office hours. Between 25% and 30% of callers will be referred to an ED. A family physician taking after-hours telephone calls may be able to limit referrals to an ED to only 10% to 20% of calls. So physicians in a strict managed care environment should ask the telephone triage nurse to handle all calls, but those calls for which the guidelines recommend an ED referral should be passed on to the physician for further triage.

Acknowledgment

I am grateful to Bill King, PhD, at Alabama Children's Hospital, for his help in working out the details about compensation of nurses.

Chapter 23

After-Hours Telephone Care: Determining and Implementing the Best Options for Your Practice

This chapter describes several options that can be used by practices to handle after-hours telephone care. The data on call volumes and distribution come from studies conducted in Colorado practices and may not accurately reflect those in your setting. They can, however, serve as examples for calculating staffing needs and budgetary implications. Each of the 5 scenarios includes sample practice objectives, call volumes, staffing options, and a budget.

Choosing the Best After-Hours Telephone Triage and Advice Options for Your Practice

There are a variety of options for handling after-hours telephone triage and advice.

- Physician on call
- Mid-level practitioner on call
- Nurse on call
- Medical call center
- Service bureau
- Combinations

There are several considerations in deciding which options are best for you.

- Expense—Using service bureaus is the most expensive option. Then, in order of expense: medical call centers, mid-level practitioners, and nurses. Least expensive are on-call physicians. But what is the actual expense to the physician of working those long overnight hours? It really cannot be quantified.
- Quality of care—The quality of care has never been adequately compared among these options. In mock call tests, mid-level practitioners always score better than physicians. Nurses using guidelines perform better than those who do not use them. Physicians generally agree with decisions made by nurses using guidelines, but are willing and able to more aggressively manage after-hours care. There have been no studies of actual outcomes.
- Availability—The number of medical call centers has been decreasing. The willingness of mid-level practitioners and nurses to take after-hours calls varies from community to community. In many communities, there is a shortage of nurses.
- Developmental stage of the provider and practice—Physicians in new practices may be more willing to take after-hours calls early in their career. Physicians in competitive environments also may be more willing to do so. Many established physicians find themselves willing to exchange income for quality of life. Providers must decide what is best for them personally.
- Quality of life for the physician—It has been shown that delegating after-hours telephone coverage lengthens the practice life of a physician by as much as 10 years. Spouses report that it also dramatically improves family life. This must be balanced with financial considerations.

The following 5 scenarios are the ones most commonly selected by family practices. Decisions about after-hours telephone care coverage are dependent on very personal preferences and objectives; and, just a reminder—your decision making will be enhanced if you collect your own data to assist in selecting the option that will work best for your practice.

1. Nurse Coverage of All After Hours

Scenario: There are 5 family practices in the city, with a total of 25 family physicians among them. A general hospital in another city is willing to provide after-hours telephone care for $15 per call. There are plenty of new patients in town, and the practices are booming. The physicians have decided to band together to develop a nurse triage system for their 5 practices.

Objective: Delegate all after-hours call coverage to office nurses from the 5 practices.

Call volumes and staffing decisions: The first step is to keep track of after-hours calls for several weeks to estimate call volumes. Then, call volumes for other seasons can be estimated (summer volumes = winter volumes x 0.65). (If you are unable to obtain data, use estimates in Table 22-1 in Chapter 22.) Usually, one triage nurse can handle the calls of 25 family physicians during all after hours (Table 22-2 in Chapter 22). Nurses can provide the after-hours call coverage from one of the offices or from home. Each nurse is given a copy of the telephone care guidelines and the supplies described in Chapter 10. Using data from the practices, the physicians estimate they will receive around 15,000 after-hours calls per year as follows: 25 calls per weeknight and 45 to 50 per weekend day and night in the summer and 40 calls per weeknight and 75 to 80 per weekend day and night in the winter. Approximately 85% of the calls will come in before 11:00 pm. They estimate that the nurse will be able to handle 8 to 9 calls per hour.

Case #1	
Expenses	**Budget**
Operating expenses	
Personnel	$68,188 [$4.55 per call]
Pay to outside service	$0
Supplies	$200 [$0.01 per call]
Subtotal	$68,388
Capital costs	
Books	$900
Furniture	$0
Subtotal	$900
Total expenses, first year	$69,288 [$4.62 per call]
Income	
Reimbursement	$0
Margin	-$69,288 [-$2,772 per physician]

Budget: The nurses in these practices typically earn $16 an hour (plus an additional $3 in benefits per hour) during the day and have agreed to a $4 differential for working nights, for a total compensation of $23 per hour for night triage and advice. The nurses also have agreed to being compensated on a per-call basis during peak hours of $3.75. After intense negotiation about calls after 11:00 pm, they agreed to a base pay of $25 for 11:00 pm to 7:00 am, plus $5 per call.

At those rates, 85% of calls will be compensated at $3.75 per call and 15% of calls will be compensated at $5 per call, plus $25 per shift. Total nursing compensation will be a little more than $68,000 for the year, or approximately $4.55 per call. Almost all of the other expenses are already being paid by the offices (eg, supplies, answering service, fixed office expenses). Incremental supplies and resource materials cost roughly $200 a year. At present, there is no reimbursement for nurses providing telephone care, so no income will be generated.

These physicians are willing to pay nearly $2,800 per year to avoid handling night calls, and the nurses welcome the additional income.

2. Medical Call Center Coverage of All After Hours

Scenario: A 7-physician family practice has decided to stop taking all night calls and use a local general hospital call center instead. The medical call center charges $6.50 per call. The practice does not have many managed care contracts and is not interested in second-level triage.

Objective: The physicians want to avoid after-hours call coverage by using a medical call center for all after-hours calls.

Call volumes and staffing decisions: The first step is to keep track of call volumes for several weeks. Then, estimate volumes in other seasons (summer volumes = winter volumes x 0.65). (If you are unable to obtain data, use estimates in Table 22-1 in Chapter 22.) Using their own practice data, the physicians estimate 5,000 after-hours calls per year. The practice should evaluate the medical call center as described in Chapter 21 and its after-hours telephone triage and advice guidelines as described in Chapter 3. The physicians need to take responsibility for educating the answering service about advising callers with nonclinical concerns to call during regular practice hours.

Budget: Because the practice estimates 5,000 calls over the year, the anticipated cost will be $32,500, or $4,643 per physician in the practice. Some time will be spent by the office staff filing the reports received from the medical call center each morning. Because the physicians were documenting after-hours calls, this is not a new function. At present,

Case #2	
Expenses	**Budget**
Operating expenses Personnel Pay to outside service Supplies	 $0 $32,500 [$6.50 per call] $0
Subtotal	$32,500
Capital costs Books and supplies Furniture	 $0 $0
Subtotal	$0
Total expenses, first year	$32,500 [$6.50 per call]
Income Reimbursement	 $0
Margin	-$32,500 [-$4,643 per physician]

there is no reimbursement for nurses providing telephone care, so no income will be generated.

3. Combination: Physician Coverage of Peak Hours and Medical Call Center Coverage of Nonpeak Hours

Scenario: An urban 7-physician family practice has access to a good medical call center that charges $12 a call, but the practice has decided that charge is more than it can afford (coverage for all after-hours calls would cost $8,571 per physician per year, or $60,000 for the practice per year). The physicians' primary objective is to get sleep at night, so they are willing to pay for the medical call center for nonpeak hours.

Objective: The physicians are willing to handle their peak after-hours calls and to pay for the medical call center for nonpeak hours to be able to sleep after 11:00 pm.

Call volumes and staffing decisions: Keep track of call volumes for several weeks. Then, estimate volumes in other seasons (summer volumes = winter volumes x 0.65). (If you are unable to obtain data, use estimates in Table 22-1 in Chapter 22.) Using its own data, the practice estimates 5,000 after-hours calls a year. Of those, roughly 85% will be prior to 11:00 pm (4,250) and handled by the physicians in the practice. So, approximately 750 calls will be managed by the medical call center. The practice should evaluate the medical call center as described in Chapter 21 and its after-hours telephone triage and advice guidelines as described in Chapter 3. It needs to take responsibility for educating the answering service about advising callers with nonclinical concerns.

Case #3	
Expenses	**Budget**
Operating expenses Personnel Pay to outside service Supplies	$0 $9,000 [$12 per call] $0
Subtotal	$9,000
Capital costs Books and supplies Furniture	$0 $0
Subtotal	$0
Total expenses, first year	$9,000 [$12 per call]
Income Reimbursement	$28,000*
Margin†	-$9,000 [-$1,286 per physician]

*If the physicians decide to charge for their telephone care, the income (theoretically, $28,000 is possible) should more than cover the cost of the medical call center.

†Without factoring in reimbursement.

Budget: Because it estimates that 750 calls will be managed by the medical call center at an expense of $12 a call, it expects to pay $9,000 for this service per year. Some time will be spent by the office staff filing the reports that have been faxed from the medical call center each morning. Because its physicians were documenting after-hours calls, this is not a new function. At present, there is no reimbursement for nurses providing telephone care. There is some reimbursement for physicians providing clinical care by telephone. If the practice decides to charge, it is possible to obtain 33% reimbursement. Theoretically (not including the expense of billing), it is possible that physicians could be reimbursed $28,000 (4,250 calls x $20 per call x 33% reimbursement rate). If the physicians are successful in charging for the telephone care they provide, the net expense per physician would drop from $5,285 to $1,286 per year per physician in the practice.

4. Combination: Nurse Coverage of Peak After Hours and Medical Call Center Coverage of Nonpeak Hours

Scenario: A 5-physician family practice wants to eliminate night call coverage. There are 5 practices in the city, for a total of 25 physicians. All 5 practices are willing to work together. A general hospital in another city is willing to provide after-hours telephone care for $12 per call, but the physicians cannot afford to pay this amount for all calls.

Objective: The physicians are willing to set up a nurse triage system using their office nurses during peak after hours. Then, they will have nonpeak hours covered by the medical call center.

Call volumes and staffing decisions: Keep track of call volumes for several weeks. Then, estimate volumes in other seasons (summer volumes = winter volumes x 0.65). (If you are unable to obtain data, use estimates in Table 22-1 in Chapter 22.) Using their data, the practices estimate 15,000 after-hours calls per year for all of the physicians in town. Of those, roughly 85% will be prior to 11:00 pm (nearly 12,750) and handled by the telephone nurses in the practices. Roughly 2,250 calls will be managed by the medical call center. The nurses will be covering peak hours, which equal 63 hours a week, and paid $3.75 per call (as in option 1). It is anticipated that one nurse will be able to handle all calls at any given time. The practices should evaluate the medical call center as described in Chapter 21 and their after-hours telephone triage and advice guidelines as described in Chapter 3. The practices need to take responsibility for educating the answering service about advising callers with nonclinical concerns.

Case #4	
Expenses	**Budget**
Operating expenses Personnel Pay to outside service Supplies	 $47,812.50 [$3.75 per call] $27,000 [$12 per call] $0
Subtotal	$74,812.50 [$4.99 per call]
Capital costs Books and supplies Furniture	 $900 $0
Subtotal	$900
Total expenses, first year	$75,712.50 [$5.05 per call]
Income Reimbursement	 $0
Margin	-$75,712.50 [-$3,028.50 per physician]

Budget: Because they estimate that 12,750 calls will be managed by the practice nurses at an expense of $3.75 a call, they expect to pay $47,812.50 to their nurses over the year. The medical call center will charge $12 a call for approximately 2,250 calls, for a total of $27,000. The overall cost is just about $5 per call and a little more than $3,000 per physician. Some time will be spent by the office staff filling in the office medical records and the reports that have been faxed from the medical call center each morning. Because the physicians were documenting after-hours calls, this is not a new function. At present, there is no reimbursement for nurses providing telephone care, so no income will be generated.

5. Combination: Nurse Coverage of Peak After Hours and Physician Coverage of Nonpeak Hours

Scenario: A 7-physician family practice in a rural area does not have access to a medical call center, but the physicians want relief from peak hours telephone calls so the physicians can more comfortably and efficiently handle the after-hours obstetric care, newborn care, inpatient care, nursing home coverage, and emergency department care. Its office nurses are willing to handle peak after-hours calls.

Objective: The office nurses will handle peak after-hours calls and the physicians will handle calls after 11:00 pm.

Call volumes and staffing decisions: The practice estimates 5,000 calls per year for the 7 physicians, of which 85% (4,250) will be peak hours and handled by the nurses and 15% (750) will be handled during non-peak hours by the on-call physicians. The nurses agreed to the compensation described in option 4.

Case #5	
Expenses	**Budget**
Operating expenses	
Personnel	$15,937.50 [$3.75 per call]
Pay to outside service	$0
Supplies	$0
Subtotal	$15,937.50 [$3.75 per call]
Capital costs	
Books and supplies	$900
Furniture	$0
Subtotal	$900
Total expenses, first year	$16,837.50 [$3.96 per call]
Income	
Reimbursement	$5,000*
Margin	-$11,837.50 [$-1,691 per physician]

*Theoretically, if the physicians decide to charge for their telephone care, the revenue generated could cover about one third of the cost of the nurse triage.

Budget: The nurses will handle roughly 4,250 calls at $3.75 per call, for a cost of $15,937.50 per year. The physicians will handle the 750 nonpeak calls a year, an average of about 2 calls per night. Theoretically, with a 33% reimbursement rate, the physicians could collect about $5,000 for this care. Other options can be explored using this method. The option that is best for your practice depends on your specific needs and objectives.

Adapting the Office Schedule to Reduce the Number of After-Hours Clinical Calls

When offices extend office hours into the weekday evening, or offer office hours on Saturday and Sunday mornings (or on holiday mornings), the number of clinical calls for the rest of the day or night can be reduced by 40% to 60%. So for larger practices, or during high-volume times, it may be cost-effective to have extended office hours, and it may reduce the after-hours call volumes as well.

Appendix A

Checklists for Getting Started

Telephone Care During Office Hours

☐ Select the team that will plan and implement your telephone care system: a medical director (physician or mid-level practitioner) for telephone care in the practice (Chapter 1), a telephone care manager (Chapter 1), and the office manager (or someone representing a business perspective).

☐ Each team member will read the manual (or the telephone care manager can read all chapters and the others read pertinent chapters).

☐ Select telephone care guidelines (Chapter 3).

☐ Define a model call, including specific expectations for actions and duration of each element of the call (Chapter 6).

☐ Select the support materials and design the work space. Later, adapt the work space to the needs of the individuals (Chapter 10).

☐ Define caller satisfaction standards (Chapter 11).

☐ Define performance standards based on the model call and caller satisfaction standards (Chapter 7).

☐ Design performance evaluation forms to evaluate calls by observation and to evaluate call documentation by reviewing logs (Chapter 7).

☐ Write a job description for telephone care providers (Chapter 8).

☐ Write initial policies and procedures or adapt those provided in this manual (Chapter 9).

☐ Collect data on call volume and call flow to develop a plan for staffing for telephone care (Chapter 17).

☐ Develop a plan for retaining good telephone care staff (Chapter 17).

☐ Decide how you want the system to work from a cost-containment standpoint, and make adjustments in your system (Chapter 19).

☐ Decide how you want your system to work from the caller standpoint, and write a description of what you would like the callers to know and do when they use the telephone care system in your practice (Chapter 13).

☐ Using the materials developed in the earlier steps and the appropriate chapters in this manual, organize an orientation for telephone care providers (Chapter 6).

☐ Select telephone care providers, if you do not have them already (Chapter 5).

☐ Orient and train the telephone care providers (Chapter 6).

☐ Develop and implement a complaint resolution system (Chapter 12).

☐ Develop and implement a quality improvement (QI) system (Chapter 14).

☐ Evaluate the performance of the telephone care providers regularly (Chapter 7).

☐ Evaluate the system (QI) regularly and replan and implement the new plans, initially with a short cycle and later with a longer cycle (Chapter 14).

☐ Review with the telephone care staff your plans for retention and adapt the plans to their feedback (Chapter 17).

Setting Up a System for Telephone Care After Hours Using Staff From Your Office

☐ Read this manual in its entirety.

☐ Read chapters 20 through 23 to decide the specific after-hours model you want to implement.

☐ Select the team that will plan and implement your telephone care system: a medical director (physician or mid-level practitioner) for telephone care in the practice (Chapter 1), a telephone care manager (Chapter 1), and the office manager (or someone representing a business perspective).

☐ Select telephone care guidelines (Chapter 3).

☐ Define a model call, including specific expectations for actions and duration of each element of the call (Chapter 6).

☐ Select the support materials and design the work space (in office or at home). Later, adapt the work space to the needs of the individuals (Chapter 10).

☐ Define caller satisfaction standards (Chapter 11).

☐ Define performance standards based on the model call and caller satisfaction standards (Chapter 7).

☐ Design performance evaluation forms to evaluate calls by observation and to evaluate call documentation by reviewing logs (Chapter 7).

☐ Write a job description for telephone care providers (Chapter 8).

☐ Write initial policies and procedures or adapt those provided in this manual (Chapter 9).

☐ Collect data on call volume and call flow to develop a plan for staffing for telephone care (Chapter 17).

☐ Develop a plan for retaining good telephone care staff (Chapter 17).

☐ Decide how you want the system to work from a cost-containment standpoint, and make adjustments in your system (Chapter 19).

☐ Decide how you want your system to work from the caller standpoint, and write a description of what you would like the callers to know and do when they use the telephone care system in your practice (Chapter 13).

☐ Using the materials developed in the earlier steps and the appropriate chapters in this manual, organize an orientation for telephone care providers (Chapter 6).

☐ Select telephone care providers, if you do not have them already (Chapter 5).

☐ Orient and train the telephone care providers (Chapter 6).

☐ Develop and implement a complaint resolution system (Chapter 12).

☐ Develop and implement a QI system (Chapter 14).

☐ Evaluate the performance of the telephone care providers regularly (Chapter 7).

☐ Evaluate the system (QI) regularly and replan and implement the new plans, initially with a short cycle and later with a longer cycle (Chapter 14).

☐ Review with the telephone care staff your plans for retention and adapt the plans to their feedback (Chapter 17).

Selection and Use of a Medical Call Center

☐ Read all chapters, especially chapters 20, 21, and 23 and Appendix C.

☐ Collect data on after-hours call volumes and call flow.

☐ Determine availability of medical call centers, details of their operations, and charges.

☐ Evaluate the expertise of medical call centers: guidelines, medical direction, nursing experience, training of nurses, performance evaluation process, QI process, and ongoing education of telephone care nurses.

☐ Evaluate the track record of medical call centers: caller satisfaction, subscribing physician satisfaction, adverse outcome record, complaint rate, referral for after-hours care rate, call response time. Also, talk to current subscribing physicians.

☐ Select the medical call center that best balances expertise, a good track record, and charges.

☐ Determine what hours of operation you want to use to balance your needs and the costs.

☐ Review documentation of all calls daily—communicate concerns with the medical call center and provide patient follow-up information where appropriate for educational purposes.

Appendix B

Telephone Care Training for Physicians

The focus of this appendix is on training physicians to provide high-quality telephone care, which can increase caller satisfaction, decrease liability, and improve efficiency. Despite these documented advantages, physician education on telephone management is still limited. In the past, most physicians learned to provide telephone care "on the job," without special training. Even today, fewer than half of all residencies offer formal training in telephone care, and evaluating telephone skills during residency has been difficult. One study found that primary care physicians asked fewer than 50% of the critical questions necessary for adequate triage. Telephone care training for residents and physicians who are new to practice dramatically reduces the time required to develop the necessary skills.

The 2 greatest teaching challenges of telephone care are content and communication. The spectrum of potential content for each telephone call is vast and can range from routine questions about breastfeeding to emergency management of a suicide attempt. It is daunting to consider teaching the entire range of potential content and all of the questions needed to evaluate it. The second factor relates to the inherent difficulty of teaching communication skills. Because telephone interactions rely solely on verbal cues without visual aids, excellent communication skills become even more important to a successful telephone interchange than for an office visit. Communication skills are notoriously difficult to teach as well as evaluate.

Teaching the New Family Physician in Your Practice

Whether physicians or nurses are providing telephone care, many elements of a successful call are universal, such as organization of the call, standardization and comprehensiveness of questions, communication skills, documentation, and call closure. These topics are covered in chapters 4 and 6. However, a major difference in training nurses in telephone care and training physicians is the use of telephone guidelines. Physicians have historically resisted using standardized guidelines for a variety of reasons. Many view the guidelines as unnecessary, cumbersome, and likely to interfere with the flow of conversation. This impression usually results from initial attempts to use guidelines, but experience shows that fluidity for all providers improves rapidly with practice. There are many advantages for physicians using guidelines, including

- Medicolegal risk reduction.
- Increased organization and efficiency.
- Standardized care among practice members.
- Easier, more time-efficient documentation (can write "advice per guideline" and know what that means).
- Role modeling for other staff members.
- It is the easiest way to train a resident or new physician.

Even if a physician does not use telephone care guidelines in day-to-day practice, the most effective way to teach telephone care is to use a standardized organizational structure (the model call, Chapter 6) and standardized telephone care guidelines (Chapter 3). By following a routine path of inquiry, the conversation remains focused and all critical information can be gathered. Having a complete picture of the patient's condition facilitates making the correct triage decision and allows the advice that is given to be more pertinent and complete. Telephone care training for new physicians should focus on the material in Chapter 6 (especially the model call). Newly trained physicians should be encouraged to use telephone care guidelines for at least the first year of practice.

Call Elements

- Introduction—The physician should introduce himself or herself and his or her professional role.
- Demographics—Depending on the setting, this information can be collected by a receptionist or the physician. The physician should verify any clinical information that he or she did not personally collect.
- History—It is helpful to begin obtaining historical information by asking an open-ended question such as, "How can I help?" or "What is the problem I can help with today?" to establish the chief complaint and then progress to more specific questions. Beginning with an open-ended question allows the caller to prioritize his or her concerns and helps to establish good communication. The physician should give the caller his or her full attention and jot down notes as the caller gives pertinent information. The primary objective is to develop as full a mental picture of the patient as possible. When using standardized guidelines, the open-ended question helps the physician to determine the most appropriate guideline to use, and the guideline provides the more specific questions. After listening to the caller's response to the open-ended question, the questions should become more specific to enable the call to be focused and efficient. If guidelines are not used, the physician must be sure to ask all questions that are pertinent, including several routine questions about respiratory status, hydration, and level of activity. (See Table B-1.) Equally important to assess are questions about measures that the caller has already tried at home. The quality of the home interventions provides the physician with good clues to assess the caller's level of knowledge and experience. Lastly, a brief medical history should be obtained. Management of a patient who is vomiting takes a different turn if that patient has heart disease and is on digoxin and lasix, for example.
- Triage decision—The triage decision may be based on the telephone care guideline or experience of the physician. The physician should recognize additional factors that influence triage decisions, such as the quality of the history and proficiency demonstrated by the caller, chronic illness in the patient, and barriers to obtaining health care.
- Advice—Advice on interim care is based on the patient's triage disposition. Care advice for emergent situations might include recommendations on the mode of transportation to the emergency facility (eg, car versus ambulance). Advice for home care is often more extensive. The physician should tailor the advice to the needs of the caller based on measures that have already been tried. Appropriate home care already instituted can be reinforced, and suggestions to modify inappropriate home care can be offered.
- Closing statements—All phone calls should conclude with a follow-up plan. Most of the time the follow-up plan consists of the callback parameters. Callback parameters include

Table B-1
Useful Questions for Telephone Assessment of the Patient

These can be remembered as the "A, B, C, D, S"

A—Airway	"Is the patient struggling to breathe or making noise while breathing?"
B—Breathing	"Is the patient breathing fast or hard?"
C—Circulation	This is a measure of hydration status. "How much has the patient had to drink?" "When did he or she last urinate?" "Has the patient had vomiting or diarrhea?"
D—Deficits	"What is the patient's level of consciousness and activity?" "What is the patient's level of activity and alertness?"
S—Skin	"Does the patient have a blotchy, purple rash?"

Other critical questions include

Medical history	"Has the patient previously been healthy?" "Has the patient ever been hospitalized?" "Does the patient take any medications?"
Home management	"What have you tried already to help the patient?"

specific signs and symptoms that indicate worsening disease and a projection for the expected course of illness. The caller should be instructed to call again if the patient develops those concerning symptoms or the illness does not improve as expected. Any barriers to achieving recommended advice should be explored. The physician should assess whether the caller understands and is comfortable with the advice, is able and intends to follow the advice, and has additional questions.

• Documentation—The physician should document the call as it proceeds. All documentation should be completed at the time of the call. Complete documentation includes the demographic information, chief complaint, and critical components of the history, such as respiratory status, hydration, and level of activity. The triage disposition should be recorded (with the guideline used, if appropriate). Any significant deviations from the guideline or customary treatment should be explained. Care advice should be summarized briefly and follow-up plans recorded. This documentation can be performed with checklists, computer programs, or in narrative format as long as the documentation is clear, complete, and legible. The report should be signed, dated, and timed. Telephone care guidelines dramatically decrease documentation time because the physician simply records the name of the guideline used, lists the pertinent positive questions, and writes "advice per guideline."

Methods of Instruction

Whether the physician is a resident or new physician in the practice, chapters 2 through 4, 6, 9, 14, 16 through 20, and this appendix should be required reading. It would be quite useful for the physician to spend some time observing a skilled, experienced telephone care provider. It also would be helpful for the new physician to observe one or more experienced physicians handling telephone calls after hours. And it is even more useful for an experienced physician to observe and critique the telephone care provided by the new physician. The experienced physician can use the evaluation checklist (see Telephone Care Evaluation Form at the end of this appendix) to assist in evaluating and providing feedback. An experienced physician should review the documentation of the new physician during the early months in practice. It is highly recommended that new physicians use telephone care guidelines during the early months (or years) in practice.

Resident Education

A telephone management education program should be tailored to match the needs and resources of the residency program. The following are some recommendations for developing a telephone care training program for residents.

Use Multiple Methods of Instruction

Lecture may be better suited for introducing the basics of organizational and communication skills. Written materials are better suited for teaching content and can include standardized protocols and/or published manuals including chapters 2 through 4 and 6 of this book. Reviewing the 10 most commonly used guidelines provides a good starting point and keeps the learner from being overwhelmed by content. The "top 10" cover 50% of all incoming calls. (See Chapter 3.) The learner can review these materials prior to the educational session. A brief quiz on written materials allows the preceptor to assess how well the learner processed the information.

An educational session can begin with a brief lecture to explain background and the importance of telephone management and to introduce basic concepts such as a structured approach to organizing the telephone call, factors that influence triage decisions, the rationale for good documentation, medicolegal risk reduction, the principles of good communication, and specific techniques for dealing with difficult callers. The session can shift from theoretical to practical considerations by reviewing a transcript of a telephone interaction followed by group discussion. The call can be designed to demonstrate examples of good and bad telephone techniques. This can be followed by small-group role-playing sessions using "scripts" in which one group member takes the role of the patient, one member plays the physician, and other members complete a Telephone Care Evaluation Form while listening to the interaction. This format allows for active practice and discussion of communication skills and provides a less threatening atmosphere than live calls. The group can give feedback to its members using the structured evaluation form, which can be supplemented by the educator.

More advanced learners may begin to take calls independently with preceptor feedback afterward. The preceptor may listen to the calls directly, tape and review them later, or review written documentation. When the preceptor listens to calls or tapes them, confidentiality issues must be addressed proactively. When the preceptor reviews written documentation, it is difficult to assess organization or communication skills. Direct observation of the resident handling calls is best.

Evaluation

The resident needs evaluation and feedback to improve performance. The educator needs evaluation to gauge how well the educational goals are being met. Evaluation of telephone care requires a combination of objective and subjective evaluation measures. Conduct a complete yet efficient medical evaluation during a telephone interaction.

Evaluating "completeness" requires an objective measure such as deviation from the model call or guideline. Feedback on selection of the appropriate guideline also should be given. If no guidelines are used, the completeness of the history can be evaluated using a predetermined checklist, such as the Telephone Care Evaluation Form, derived from established guidelines or developed by group consensus. Evaluating efficiency can be accomplished by an objective measure, such as timing the length of the call.

Evaluation of communication skills requires more subjective measures. Objective measures are important to evaluate but sometimes miss the essence of the call and fail to adequately evaluate communication and organizational skills. The physician may ask all the critical questions, but may do so in a disorganized or noninteractive fashion. Advice may be given in a perfunctory manner that does not adapt to the individual situation. The objective measures can be supplemented with subjective measures to capture the success of achieving good communication skills.

The Telephone Care Evaluation Form can be used by preceptors or peers using live or simulated calls. Because telephone care skills have not traditionally been taught in residency programs, preceptors may feel uncomfortable about giving feedback. Faculty development sessions and use of structured feedback forms can address this issue.

Preceptor_____   Date_____

Resident_____

TELEPHONE CARE EVALUATION FORM

Greeting   **Comments**

_____ Did the greeting include the physician's name, title,
and offer of assistance?
_____ Was all demographic information included?
_____ Name of patient   _____ Name of caller and
_____ Age of patient   relation to child
_____ Phone number

Critical Questions

_____ Was enough information obtained to ensure stable airway
breathing?
_____ Level of consciousness and activity is appropriate?
_____ Vomiting or diarrhea?
_____ Fluid intake?
_____ Urine output?
_____ Fever?
_____ Rash?
_____ Duration of illness?
_____ Home management inquired about?

Medical History

_____ Chronic illness
_____ Prescription and nonprescription medicine

Triage

_____ Was an appropriate triage guideline selected?
_____ Was an appropriate triage decision made?

Management

_____ Was an appropriate management plan or advice given?
_____ Was the advice clear?
_____ Was the caller's understanding and ability to follow the plan verified?
_____ Was appropriate follow-up arranged (ie, a visit or parameters for
which to call and permission to call back given)?
_____ Did the physician reinforce appropriate home care already
instituted?

Communication

_____ Did the physician begin with an open-ended question?
_____ Was the tone of the physician pleasant and empathetic?
_____ Were leading questions or multiple questions used?
_____ Was the physician organized or rambling? (Circle one.)
_____ Was the call too short, too long, or just right? (Circle one.)
_____ Did the physician listen attentively and ask questions to clarify?
_____ Did the physician communicate clearly? If not, what could have

Appendix C

Evaluating Medical Call Centers

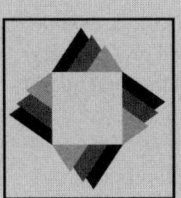

American Academy of Pediatrics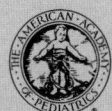

STRATEGIES FOR PRACTICE MANAGEMENT

A Report from the Provisional Section on Pediatric Telephone Care and the Committee on Practice and Ambulatory Medicine

NOVEMBER 1998

PEDIATRIC CALL CENTERS AND THE PRACTICE OF TELEPHONE TRIAGE AND ADVICE: CRITICAL SUCCESS FACTORS

There has been dramatic growth in the development and implementation of pediatric call centers. Major medical centers, insurance companies, physician groups, and other health care organizations have established pediatric call centers and they are rapidly becoming the standard of pediatric after-hours telephone care in many communities.[1,2] It is conservatively estimated that currently 25% of all general pediatricians use an after-hours call center to address their patients' needs.[1,2] The primary stimuli supporting their growth are managed care and the increased emphasis on demand management. However, the need to combine quality demand management services with efficient and productive telephone care creates a potential marketplace conflict that may lead to the practice of less than optimal, or even unsafe, telephone care.

The growth in telephone medicine was the result of several factors that emerged in the early 1990s. Changes in physician lifestyle, research demonstrating nurses' competency to perform telephone triage, growth in managed care, and the emer-

gence of vertically integrated systems of care and their reliance on demand management (eg, providing the best medical care to the most patients in the most appropriate cost-effective setting) — all contributed to the growth. In addition, health care mergers and downsizing resulted in less contact between the physician and the patient. Integrated delivery systems and managed care organizations (MCOs) structured themselves to facilitate easy access to health care services while preventing the excessive cost associated with inappropriate emergency room and urgent care center visits.

Physician report cards, the National Committee on Quality Assurance's (NCQA) Health Plan and Employer Data Information Set (HEDIS)®3.0 performance measures, the Joint Commission on the Accreditation of Healthcare Organization's (JCAHO) requirements, and the Clinical Laboratory Improvement Amendment Acts of 1988 (CLIA) mandates, and hospital quality-of-care reports have all become means to ensure the delivery of optimal patient care while contributing to the reduction in medical care costs seen in recent decades. Despite the facts that quali-

ty monitoring and standards of care have become routine in the current practice of medicine and that telephone care has been estimated to account for 12% to 27% of the practice of pediatrics,[3,4] no quality assurance guidelines have been created for medical call centers. The following monograph identifies and describes critical success factors designed to facilitate the safe and effective operation of pediatric call centers and the practice of high-quality triage and advice.

Currently there are over 50 pediatric call centers across the country; hundreds more provide pediatric and adult services. Numerous managed care and pharmaceutical companies and even national drug store chains have advice lines. It has been estimated that approximately 35 million people have access to telephone triage and advice, with the number growing exponentially.[5] For example, a 1993 study reported the success of the Denver After-Hours Program in which over 100,000 calls were answered with no reported major adverse outcome. The program obtained a 100% physician satisfaction and 96% to 99% patient satisfaction rating.[1]

1 Poole SR, Schmitt BD, Carruth T, et al. After-hours telephone coverage: the application of an area-wide telephone triage and advice system for pediatric practices. Pediatrics. 1993;92:670-679

2 Pert JC, Furth TW, Katz HP. A 10-year experience in pediatric after-hours telecommunications. Current Opinion in Pediatrics. 1996; 8:181-187

3 Bergman AB, Dassel SW, Wedgewood RJ. Time-motion study of practicing pediatricians. Pediatrics. 1966; 38:254-263

4 Hessel SJ, Haggerty RJ. General pediatrics: a study of practice in the mid 1960's. Pediatrics. 1968; 73:271-279

5 How nurses take calls and control the care of patients from afar. The Wall Street Journal. February 4, 1997

In response to this growing trend, the American Academy of Pediatrics (AAP) formed the Provisional Section on Pediatric Telephone Care. The Provisional Section is to organize the study and advancement of telephone triage and advice as it relates to patient outcomes, standards of care, and resident/physician education.

DEVELOPMENT OF GUIDELINES

In response to this national growth in pediatric call centers, clinical and administrative representatives from pediatric call centers across the country (four physicians, seven nurses, a hospital administrator, and an attorney) have collectively developed these guidelines for the administration and management of pediatric call centers. Telephone triage and advice standards for nursing practice have been established,[6] and recently standards for the accreditation of call centers associated with managed care organizations (MCOs) have been proposed.[7] As the number of call centers increases nationally, there is a need to establish guidelines that will hold providers and call centers accountable for providing timely access to care in an appropriate setting without compromising quality and, more importantly, patient safety. These guidelines are intended to provide a comprehensive outline for the safe operation of pediatric call centers and to form a framework for the development of standards of care.

These guidelines are divided into five sections: call center operations, patient access, nursing, physician interaction, and total quality management. The drafts were reviewed by staff of 12 pediatric call centers, members of the American Association of Ambulatory Care Nursing and members of the AAP Provisional Section on Pediatric Telephone Care and the Committee on Medical Liability.

PEDIATRIC CALL CENTER DEFINITION

A pediatric call center provides health care management to patients whose primary care provider practices within the broad scope of pediatrics. These providers include pediatricians, nurse practitioners, and general and family physicians. Services provided by the call center may include, but are not limited to, telephone triage and advice, physician referral, scheduling, utilization management, and disease and wellness management. Pediatric call centers do not routinely provide Emergency Medical Services (EMS). Pediatric call centers practicing telephone triage and advice use trained registered nurses to provide the systematic assessment of patient's needs through the use of standardized protocols, algorithms, or guidelines. Call centers may act as physician representatives or operate for the benefit of the general public or specific health care organizations.

CALL CENTER OPERATIONS

A. Personnel Structure

The call center's personnel structure provides a framework within which telephone triage and advice is performed. The structure should include a medical director, clinical (nurse) administrator, and call center registered nurses.

Medical Director

The pediatric call center organization structure should include a board-certified/board-eligible pediatrician acting as the medical director. If a pediatrician is not available to function as the medical director, there should be one available to serve as a consultant. The medical director will be responsible for and oversee the clinical operation of the call center. More specifically, the medical director will write — or review — and approve all triage and advice guidelines/protocols, prescription/nonprescription medication policies, and, any policies and procedures that ensure the safe practice of telephone triage and advice, and oversee the training of the nursing staff. The medical director also will act as a physician liaison to physician and health care organization subscribers and will oversee the total quality management programs.

Clinical Nurse Administrator

The clinical nurse administrator is responsible for establishing and approving nursing policies and job descriptions and managing the nursing staff needed to support the call center. He or she also is responsible for the overall operation of the call center, including staff selection, training, scheduling, and performance evaluations, maintenance of all call processing, and the implementation of the total quality management programs.

Call Center Registered Nurse

The call center nurse will provide patient care that ensures the health, safety, and comfort of patients. This is accomplished through health education in disease prevention and management and referral to appropriate medical care. The call center nurse performs symptom-based triage guided by clinical algorithms, guidelines and/or protocols, and policies and procedures. Following these nursing resources, the call center nurse has to interpret, clarify, prioritize, differentiate, discern, and integrate clinical information to make a triage decision as to whether the child needs to be seen immediately, urgently, or for a scheduled appointment, or whether the child and/or patient needs advice about home care management or other dispositions.

Other Personnel

Call centers may utilize the following personnel to improve nurse productivity

---

TABLE 1
Policies and Procedures Related to Risk Management

- Communication with minors
- Noncompliant callers
- Angry callers
- Obscene callers
- Inability to make contact with the caller/patient (eg, wrong numbers, no answer, line busy and identified or unidentified answering machines)
- Anonymous and noncontracted callers
- Hearing and speech impaired callers and foreign language callers
- Back-up systems for technological (power or equipment) failure, natural disasters and, if computerized, process for how and when to initiate manual calls
- Nurse medication prescribing patterns in accordance with state laws
- Access to Emergency Medical Services (EMS) and Emergency Medical Services for Children (EMS-C)
- Confidentiality
- Documentation
- Nursing boundaries of practice Out-of-state calls

---

6 Telephone Nursing Practice, Administration, and Practice Standards. American Academy of Ambulatory Care Nursing. Pitman, NJ: A.J. Janetti, Inc.,1997.

7 24 Hour Telephone Triage and Health Information Standards (Draft). American Accreditation Health Care Commission/URAC. Washington, DC: 1998.

and assure optimal quality: medical advisory committee, non-clinical manager, clerical and technical support staff, and nurses with expanded roles such as supervisor or education coordinator.

B. Policies and Procedures

Nursing policies and procedures are necessary to assist the practice and refine the judgment of the telephone triage nurse and ensure the appropriate application of established guidelines/protocols. The management of calls that are not covered by clinical guidelines/protocols need to be defined through policies and procedures.

Managing Risk

Nursing policies and procedures should outline the potential risk management issues that relate to the patient care population served by the call center. Table 1 identifies key policies and procedures that need to be in place.

Assisting the Triage Process

Policies and procedures that are identified in Table 2 should be used to assist with the triage process.

C. Nursing Resources

When registered nurses accept the responsibility of providing telephone triage, they assume a specialized nursing role. To assist them in performing this function in a safe and efficient manner, nurses should have access to the following medical and nursing resources: clinical triage guidelines/protocols, printed references, physician consultations, medical laboratories, pharmacies, and community resources.

Clinical Triage Guidelines/Protocols

Triage guidelines/protocols in printed and/or computerized format should be available to help the telephone nurse provide triage and advice. Triage guidelines/protocols should cover a large majority of incoming calls about ill or injured children. All triage guidelines/protocols should contain standard referral criteria (dispositions) and standard treatment advice for managing symptoms at home. Triage guidelines/protocols should be used on all calls for which they are available. Finally, the triage guidelines/protocols should undergo the following review process:

1. Triage guidelines/protocols are initially written or reviewed, modified as necessary for local or regional standard of care, and authorized by the call center's medical director and/or advisory committee.
2. Triage guidelines/protocols are reviewed, updated as necessary, expanded and reauthorized at least yearly by the medical director and/or medical advisory committee.
3. Triage guidelines/protocols are available for optional review by subscribing primary care providers or health care organizations.

Printed References

A Reference Library present within the call center should contain pertinent texts and books about pediatric health care.

Physician Consultation

Primary care providers (PCPs) contracting with the pediatric call center for telephone triage and advice should make themselves, or a physician designee on-call, available in a timely manner to the telephone triage nurse and/or answering service for any questions regarding their patients. In addition, the medical director, or his/her clinical designee, should be on-call and available in a timely manner to the telephone triage nurse for consultation.

Medical Laboratories

If guidelines/protocols contain recommendations for ordering laboratory studies (eg, throat cultures or tests to determine bilirubin levels), the process should be standardized. These guidelines/protocols should contain clear indications for laboratory referral, telephone numbers for laboratory sites, and instructions for dealing with test results.

Pharmacies

If guidelines/protocols or related nursing policies contain recommendations for ordering new prescriptions and/or prescription refills, the process should be standardized.

Community Resources

A description of relevant services provided, hours of operation, and the telephone numbers for emergency community services should be available. Telephone numbers should be included for the call center's geographic area of coverage. These resources should include but are not limited to the following:

- Emergency medical transport
- Child protective services
- Infectious disease contacts and exposure (Public Health Department)
- Police department
- Poison center
- Sexual assault and rape crisis

resource(s)

D. Documentation

Documentation is the concise, factual record of a patient call. Documentation assists with continuity of care, quality assessment, and improvement, and it serves as the medical record of the telephone call.

Symptom-based Triage

All symptom-based triage should be documented utilizing a call form to be completed manually or a computerized reporting system and should include the registration, clinical, and, when indicated, medical information listed in Table 3.

In situations in which no patient or caller contact is made, documentation should include whether a message was left on an identified or unidentified answering machine, the time attempted call(s) was made with no answer, and/or the time an attempted call(s) was made with a busy signal.

If the call center staff initiates a follow-up call, the documentation should include the patient's current health status and any change in care advice or disposition.

TABLE 2
Policies and Procedures to Assist the Triage Process

- Multiple symptom calls
- "No Protocol" calls (calls that do not fit into an existing protocol/guideline)
- Overrides of medical guidelines/recommendations
- Medications (new prescriptions, refill prescriptions, and over-the-counter or OTC medications)
- Laboratory tests
- Suspected child abuse calls (eg, physical abuse, sexual abuse, neglect, etc.)
- Ingestions/poisonings calls
- Sexual assault calls
- Suicide calls/psychiatric-behavior management emergencies
- Chronic illness calls
- 911/emergency calls
- Procedure for telephone triage/advice, referral, and follow-up for patients with non-contracting primary care providers (PCPs) or no PCP
- Procedure for making referrals (eg, after-hours site notifications, physician referral)
- Prioritizing incoming calls

Archive of Records

All telephone encounter documentation should be archived.

PATIENT ACCESS TO CALL CENTER

Universal access to the call center should be available to all patients enrolled in a subscribing physician's practice or contracting organization. Patients should be informed of the relationship between the organization/practice and the call center to ensure continuity of care and patient and physician satisfaction.

A. Overall Access

All patients enrolled in a practice or organization that offers a telephone triage and advice service should have access to that service regardless of insurance, socioeconomic status, disabilities, age or communication problems, providing the patient/family has access to a telephone.

B. Patient Notification

Pediatric call centers, acting in their role as patient advocates, should advise all subscribing practices and organizations to inform and educate their enrolled patients regarding the triage and advice program.

C. Access to Telephone Triage Nursing Staff

Patients should have access to the pediatric call center's staff during contracted service hours through a telephone connection via the practice's or organization's telephone line, through an answering service, or by a direct telephone line to the call center. All callers should be informed immediately of the status (name and role) of the staff member with whom they are speaking (eg, first name, job title, etc).

NURSING

A. Education, Licensure, and Clinical Competency

The telephone triage nurse should be a graduate of an approved nursing program and should hold RN licensure according to state laws. The telephone triage nurse should have experience in pediatric nursing or telephone nursing experience with pediatric patients. Nurses with experience that is not pediatric-based should undergo extensive pediatric education and training and work under the supervision of a pediatric-trained nurse. When available, telephone triage nurses should strive for certification.

The telephone triage nurse should demonstrate competency in Communication and technical skills and should be able to function automonously using the nursing process, critical thinking, assessment and problem-solving skills, and good clinical judgment.

B. Training

Specialty training and continuing education is essential to the success of telephone triage nursing, an area in which nurses do not rely on their vision or sense of touch, but are heavily dependent on a blend of traditional nursing and extensive assessment and communication skills. The orientation and training program should include the teaching and evaluation of nurses on technical and communication skills, call center operations (including details of available nursing resources and nursing policies and procedures), the nursing process as it relates to telephone triage and advice (see Table 4), call processing, and the skills needed to function autonomously. Specific instruction should be given on the importance of proper documentation and other pertinent patient care and risk management issues. It is essential to the safe practice of pediatric telephone triage and advice that child development, wellness and disease be taught and that knowledge in these areas be assessed in the training program.

C. Nursing Clinical Competency

A periodic assessment of telephone triage nurse clinical competency should be performed. The components of clinical competency should include, but not be limited to, clinical judgment, appropriate application of the nursing process, and knowledge of boundaries of practice and accurate documentation.

D. Continuing Education

The telephone triage nurse should demonstrate self-directed and/or continu-

---

TABLE 3
Documentation Items

I. Registration Information
- Date and time of telephone call
- Name of nurse
- Name of patient (unless call is anonymous)
- Name of caller (unless call is anonymous)
- Name of PCP
- Patient's date of birth (and calculated age)

II. Clinical Information
- Presenting problem/symptom
- Nursing assessment
- Relevant medical history and current medications.
- Relevant allergies.
- Guideline/protocol or reference used.
- Advice given (health education given).
- Disposition recommended.
- Evaluation of patient's/caller's understanding of care instructions and recommended disposition.
- Evaluation of patient's/caller's intended action including follow-up.
- Physician contact.

III. Medication Information
- Prescription and OTC medication instructions: dosage, route of administration, frequency, and duration when indicated
- Patient age
- Stated patient weight
- Medication allergies
- Other medication taken by the patient

TABLE 4
Suggested call-processing sequence

Assessment
- Receive, pre-triage, and prioritize calls
- Conduct assessment interview: history of present problem, relevant past medical history, recent prior calls if available

Identification
- Identify primary problem/symptom
- Identify emergency/high-risk situations

Triage
- Select appropriate protocol/guideline or nursing resource
- Continue assessment interview
- Determine recommended disposition

Intervention
- Provide clinical care advice and education

Evaluation
- Evaluate caller's understanding of advice
- Evaluate caller's potential for compliance

Conclusion
- Consult PCP, refer, or arrange follow-up as indicated

ing education specific to the area of pediatric and telephone nursing.

E. Boundaries of Practice

The telephone triage nurse should engage in a symptom-based practice, using the nursing process and resources approved by the medical director. Each nurse also should function within the boundaries of their license and their state's Nurse Practice Act.

It is important to stress that employee records should include documentation of nursing education, licensure, pediatric experience, and training and performance evaluation.

PHYSICIAN INTERACTION

Pediatric call centers act on behalf of and in contractual agreement with physicians, their practices, and/or health care organizations. Physicians or health care organizations using call center services are ultimately responsible for the triage and advice given to their patients.[8] In order to ensure appropriate care for their patients, physicians and health care organizations have obligations to the pediatric call center. These obligations ensure the delivery of safe telephone triage and advice and enhance continuity of care for the patient.

A. Contracts

Each physician or health care organization using the services of the call center should have a contract outlining the services provided and their obligations to the center. Contracts may include statements regarding physician's or health care organization's agreement to use the triage and advice protocols and pertinent additions prior to their use by the call center. In order to ensure prompt attention to the patient's need for physician assessments and second-level triage, contracts also should delineate a reasonable time period in which physicians should return pages from the call center. The mechanism for communication between the call center and the subscribing physician or health care organization, in regard to both verbal communication and the telephone encounter document, should be stated clearly in the contract.

B. Communication

To ensure that clinical issues are addressed in a timely fashion and to guarantee patient continuity of care, it is essential that the physician and call center communicate effectively and efficiently.

A physician representing a subscribing practice should be on-call and available at all times that the call center is covering for that practice in order to assist in clinical situations that include but are not limited to the following:

- In situations when callers are insistent upon speaking with the physician directly.
- In cases when the health questions go beyond the ability, the comfort level, or the resources available to the nurse taking the call. These may include cases outside the range of clinical guidelines/protocols or children with chronic diseases or other special needs.
- The physician may elect to be contacted for certain acuity levels (eg, see immediately, etc).

- In situations when a nurse believes a caller will not comply with the recommended disposition.

C. Disposition Notification to Physician Practices

Call centers should notify subscribing physicians of the clinical disposition of all calls by the next business day, if not sooner.

TOTAL QUALITY MANAGEMENT

All call centers should have in place a total quality management program that includes quality assessment, quality assurance, and quality improvement initiatives. These programs should monitor the quality and identify deficits related to the clinical and financial aspects of the call center. Established programs should be designed to monitor at least the specific following items.

A. Call Response Time

It is essential to the practice of safe telephone triage and advice that all patient

---

TABLE 5
Call Priority Definitions

Emergent calls include, but are not limited to, calls about the following:
- Difficulty breathing (e.g., choking, stopped breathing, weak breathing, stridor, cyanosis, or other signs of respiratory distress)
- Possible anaphylaxis (difficulty breathing or swallowing following medicine, bee sting, food, or other possible allergen)
- Neurological symptom (eg, seizure, loss of consciousness, hard to awaken, confusion, altered mental status, stiff neck)
- Poisoning, ingestion, drug overdose
- Foreign body — in the airway (choking) or swallowed
- Trauma of the neck or eye
- Electric shock
- Near drowning
- Suicide — threats or attempts

Urgent calls include, but are not limited to, calls about the following:
- Trauma other than neck or eye
- Asthma, wheezing, or croup with no mention of difficulty breathing
- Foreign body — ear, nose, or vagina
- Bleeding (active) including blood in vomit or stool
- Burns except sunburn
- Bites (eg, animal, snake, spider, marine animal, bee, yellow jacket — not insects or ticks)
- Fever over 105°F
- Infant less than 3 months of age with fever
- Severe pain, especially abdomen, head, or chest
- Possible dehydration
- Purple or blood-colored rash
- Heat exhaustion or stroke
- Hypothermia
- Psychosocial emergencies (sexual assault, child abuse, domestic violence)

---

8 Policy on phone counseling. American Medical Association Report of the Board of Trustees (A-96). Chicago: 1997

calls be answered in a timely manner, appropriate to the severity of the reason for calling. Clearly, the level of severity can not be assessed fully until a nursing assessment has been performed. Therefore, determination of the urgency of the call should be based on the presenting problem as stated by the patient/caller and the guidelines suggested in Table 5.

Potentially Emergent

Patients with symptoms that indicate an immediate life-threatening illness or injury should be instructed at the point of first contact with the call center to contact their local emergency medical services (EMS) or their emergency medical services for children (EMS-C) or, if EMS is not available, have immediate access to the call center's triage services.

Potentially Urgent

Patients with symptoms that indicate illness or injuries that could deteriorate into life-threatening situations should have priority access to the call center.

Non-urgent

Patients with symptoms that indicate a delay in care would not result in life-threatening situation should have access to the call center within a reasonable amount of time.

B. Caller Access

Call centers utilizing the inbound call method (automated call distribution lines with a patient initiated call) should keep records of abandonment and blockage rates.

C. Patient/Physician/Medical Care Organization Satisfaction

Patient/caller and physician/medical care organization satisfaction should be evaluated periodically, using a statistically significant sample of callers.

D. Clinical Guidance and Resource Use Appropriateness

Call encounter documents should be reviewed for appropriate triage guideline or nursing resource selection.

E. Disposition Appropriateness

Call encounter documents should be reviewed for appropriate caller disposition and overall disposition rates should be evaluated routinely.

F. Clinical Outcomes

Call centers are encouraged to investigate routinely the clinical outcomes of care provided to patients. Outcomes analysis should demonstrate reasonable health and functional status of patients. No adverse events resulting from a delay in diagnosis or treatment should occur. Call centers also should be encouraged to monitor "see-immediately" referral rates and evaluate for unnecessary health care utilization patterns.

CONCLUSION

The use of pediatric call centers performing nurse telephone triage and advice is growing rapidly and has become the standard of care in many regions of the country. These operational and clinical practice guidelines have been developed to ensure the safe and effective operation of pediatric call centers and the practice of optimal telephone triage and advice. These guidelines pertain to the operation of a pediatric call center representing subscribing physicians and health care organizations. They are intended to be used by call centers at all levels of development, from the initial planning stage to the experienced fully operational call center.

These guidelines are based on current knowledge and data pertaining to the operation of pediatric call centers and the delivery of telephone triage and advice. They will undergo modification and clarification as clinical benchmarks are identified and evaluated and as research into this burgeoning field is performed. Specific benchmark figures have been purposely omitted from this monograph since to date no formal evaluations identifying benchmarks with outcomes or quality significance have been performed. Comments, suggestions, and collaborative data related to the topics listed in the total quality management section are strongly encouraged to guarantee the future integrity and relevance of these guidelines.

These guidelines can not be applied in entirety to the practice of office-based telephone triage and advice since the level of physician involvement and triage goals may be significantly different in an office setting. However, it is encouraged that these guidelines be used as a cornerstone for the future establishment of office-based telephone care guidelines. Through the application of these and subsequent guidelines, safe and quality patient care will always be the foremost goal and will not be compromised by managed care and financial pressures.

Provisional Section on Pediatric Telephone Care Steering Committee
- Steven R. Poole, MD, Chairperson
- Ben Gitterman, MD (Author)
- Andrew Hertz, MD (Author)
- Allison Kempe, MD, MPH
- Sanford Metzer, MD
- Hanna Sherman, MD (Author)

Committee on Practice and Ambulatory Medicine
- Jack T. Swanson, MD, Chairperson
- Edward O. Cox, MD
- F. Lane France, MD (SVM)
- Katherine C. Teets Grimm, MD
- James W. Herbert, MD
- E. Susan Hodgson, MD
- Allan S. Lieberthal, MD
- Kyle Yasuda, MD

Liaisons
- Todd Davis, MD, Ambulatory Pediatric Association
- Robert D. Chessin, MD, Section on Administration & Practice Management
- Robert Sayers, MD, Uniformed Services Section
- Emmanuel E. Eugenio, MD, Resident Section

Contributing Authors
- Sherri Cotilla, RN
- Mary DeBarr, RN
- Carol A. DiVella, RN
- Jacquelyn Kopet-Feller, PNP
- Maureen Leahy, MBA, MPH
- Patricia Best Reisinger, MS, RN
- Barton D. Schmitt, MD, FAAP
- Carol M. Stock, MN, RN, JD
- Sissy Tubb, RN, CPN
- Kathi Webster, RN

Appendix D

References in Family Medicine Literature on Telephone Care

Journal Articles and Papers

General

American Academy of Pediatrics. Pediatric Call Centers and the practice of telephone triage and advice: critical success factors. In: American Academy of Pediatrics. *Strategies for Practice Management: A Report From the Provisional Section on Pediatric Telephone Care and the Committee on Practice and Ambulatory Medicine.* Elk Grove Village, IL: American Academy of Pediatrics; 1998:1–6

Curtis P, Talbot A. The telephone in primary care. *J Community Health.* 1981;6:194–203

Darling WD, Henderson DM. *Determining Legal Pitfalls When Promoting Medical Advice.* Southborough, MA: International Business Communications; 1997

Daugird AJ, Spencer DC. Characteristics of patients who highly utilize telephone medical care in private practice. *J Fam Pract.* 1989;29:59–63

Dershewitz R. Telephone triage: time for the bell to stop tolling. *Public Health Reports.* 1980;95:326–327

Dunn JM. Warning: giving telephone advice is hazardous to your professional health. *Nursing.* August 1985;15:40–41

Fischer PM, Smith SR. The nature and management of telephone utilization in a family practice setting. *J Fam Pract.* 1979;8:321–327

Greenlick MR, Freeborn DK, Gambill GL, Pope CR. Determinants of medical care utilization: the role of the telephone in total medical care. *Med Care.* 1973;11:121–134

Hallan I. You've got a lot to answer for, Mr. Bell. A review of the use of the telephone in primary care. *J Fam Pract.* 1989;6:47–57

Henry PF. Legal principles in providing telephone advice. *Nurse Pract Forum.* September 1994;5:124–125

Katz HP, Wick W. Malpractice, meningitis, and the telephone. *Pediatr Ann.* 1991;20:85–89

Kearney KA. Legal liability and risk considerations for a medical call center. In launching and managing a medical call center. Paper presented at: National Managed Health Care Congress; 1996; Chicago, IL

Killila BA. Undocumented phone calls: a liability issue. *Indiana Med.* 1990;83:768–769

Knopke HJ, McDonald E, Silvertson SE. A study of family practice in Wisconsin. *J Fam Pract.* 1979;8:151–156

Levy JC, Rosekrans J, Lamb GA, Friedman M, Kaplan D, Strasser P. Development and field testing of protocols for the management of pediatric telephone calls: protocols for pediatric telephone calls. *Pediatrics.* 1979;64:558–563

Radecki SE, Neville RE, Girard RA. Telephone patient management by primary care physicians. *Med Care.* 1989;27:817–822

Solberg LI, Mayer TR, Seifert MH Jr, Cole PM, Holloway RL. Office telephone calls in family practice. *J Fam Pract.* 1984;18:609–613, 616

Spencer DC, Daugird AJ. The nature and content of physician telephone calls in a private practice. *J Fam Pract.* 1988;27:201–205

Sullivan G. Advice or diagnosis? A legal perspective. *Bus Health.* May 1997;15:40–42

Tammelleo AD. Staying out of trouble on the telephone. *RN.* October 1993;56:63–64

Westbury RD. The electric speaking practice: a telephone workload study. *Can Fam Physician.* 1974;20:69–76

Wheeler SQ. Telephone triage: sidestepping the pitfalls. *Nursing.* May 1994;24:32LL, 32OO

Willett DE. Medicine by telephone continued: a legal option. *Modern Med.* 1977;45:73–77

After-Hours
Bergman JJ, Rosenblatt RA. After-hours calls: a five-year longitudinal study in a family practice group. *J Fam Pract.* 1982;15:101–106

Curtis P, Talbot A, Liebeseller V. The after-hours call: a survey of United States family practice residency programs. *J Fam Pract.* 1979;8:117–122

Curtis P, Talbot A. The after-hours call in family practice. *J Fam Pract.* 1979;9:901–909

Evens S, Curtis P, Talbot A, Baer C, Smart A. Characteristics and perceptions of after-hours callers. *Fam Pract.* 1985;2:10–16

Greenhouse DL, Probst JC. After-hours telephone calls in a family practice residency: volume, seriousness, and patient satisfaction. *Fam Med.* 1995;27:525–530

Mayer TR, Solberg L, Seifert M, Cole P. After-hours telephone calls in private family practice. *J Fam Pract.* 1983;17:327–332

Perkins A, Gagnon R, deGruy F. A comparison of after-hours telephone calls concerning ambulatory and nursing home patients. *J Fam Pract.* 1993;37:247–250

Reimbursement
Melzer SM, Poole SR. Reimbursement for telephone care. *Pediatrics.* 2002;109:290–293

Books

Briggs JK. *Telephone Triage Protocols for Nurses*. 2nd ed. Philadelphia, PA: Lippincott Williams & Wilkins; 2002

Brown JL. *Pediatric Telephone Medicine: Principles, Triage, and Advice*. 2nd ed. Philadelphia, PA: Lippincott Williams & Wilkins; 1994

Brown JL. *Telephone Medicine*. Philadelphia, PA: Lippinicott Williams & Wilkins; 1980

Group Health Cooperative of Puget Sound. *Nurses' Guide to Telephone Triage & Health Care*. Baltimore, MD: Williams & Wilkins; 1985

Katz HP. *Telephone Medicine: Triage and Training for Primary Care*. 2nd ed. Philadelphia, PA: F. A. Davis Co; 2001

Long VE, McMullen PC. *Telephone Triage for Obstetrics and Gynecology*. Philadelphia, PA: Lippincott Williams & Wilkins; 2002

Schmitt BD, Baker RC. *Pediatric Telephone Advice*. 2nd ed. Philadelphia, PA: Lippincott Williams & Wilkins; 1999

Schmitt BD. *Pediatric Telephone Protocols: After-Hours Version*. 9th ed. Littleton, CO: Decision Press; 2002

Schmitt BD. *Pediatric Telephone Protocols: Office Version*. 9th ed. Elk Grove Village, IL: American Academy of Pediatrics; 2002

Swenson DE. *Telephone Triage of the Obstetric Patient: A Nursing Guide*. 2nd ed. Philadelphia, PA: WB Saunders Co; 2001

Wheeler SQ, Windt JH. *Telephone Triage: Theory, Practice, and Protocol Development*. Albany, NY: Delmar Publishers; 1993

Wheeler SQ. *Telephone Triage Protocols for Infants and Children: Birth to 6 Years*. Gaithersburg, MD: Aspen Publishers; 1997

Index